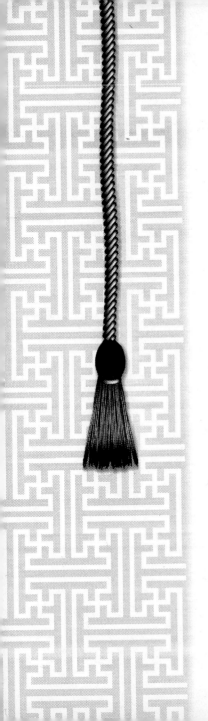

Christian Yoga
Restoration for Body & Soul

AN ILLUSTRATED GUIDE TO SELF-CARE

By Jennifer Zach
with Deanna Smothers, E-RYT
and Courtney Kutta, E-RYT

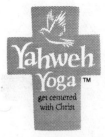

Yahweh Yoga™
get centered
with Christ

www.yahwehyoga.com

Written by Jennifer Zach, with DeAnna Smothers and Courtney Kutta; cover design by Alison King; book design by Karen Pasternack Straus; photography by Dale Kesel.

Yahweh Yoga encourages you to consult a health care professional prior to starting this or any exercise program. The publishers of this book assume no responsibility for any injury that may result from performing these exercises.

ISBN 978-1-58776-873-6
Library of Congress catalog card number: 2007941662
Manufactured in the United States of America
1 2 3 4 5 6 7 8 9 10 NetPub 0 9 8 7

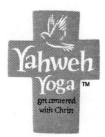

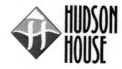

675 Dutchess Turnpike, Poughkeepsie, NY 12603
www.hudsonhousepub.com   (800) 724-1100

FOR OUR
HEAVENLY FATHER:
May this bring
you glory

✠

FOR OUR LOVED ONES:
May you be rewarded for your sacrifice and support

FOR OUR READERS: May you be blessed

✠

Dear friends,
we pray that you may
enjoy good health
and that all
may go well with you,
even as your soul is
getting along well.
3 JOHN 2

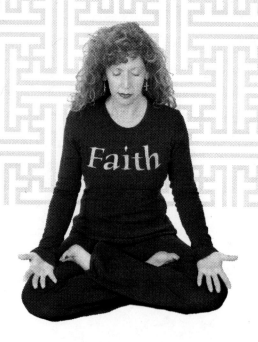

1

RESTORATION

2
SOUL

3
BODY

A Note to Our Readers

WELCOME TO YAHWEH Yoga's book *Christian Yoga: Restoration for Body and Soul*. This book was inspired by a love for the Lord and his people. As a yoga practitioner for more than 25 years I kept hearing my brothers and sisters in Christ tell me that their doctors recommended they practice yoga for their health but they were concerned that they would be practicing something that did not fit with our faith. A few years ago the Lord began whispering to me, *"Begin teaching Christian yoga."* The whisper became louder until my heart was convicted that there was nothing to do but be obedient and begin teaching Christian yoga. The rest, as they say, is history.

Yahweh Yoga is the first Christian yoga studio in the world. In its first year we have had to tear down a wall to enlarge the studio to accommodate the growing number of students coming to our classes. As an outreach we have produced several DVDs and now this beautiful book. We hope this book will be a catalyst for drawing you closer in your relationship with Christ, for taking excellent care of yourself and will encourage you that Christian yoga is indeed quite compatible with our faith.

The author of our book, Jennifer Zach, is also the Spiritual Director at Yahweh Yoga. She helps train all those wanting to become Certified Christian Yoga Teachers (CCYT) at our school. As you read her beautiful words we pray that this book will be a treasured companion to you for the renewing of your mind, body and soul. As you will discover within these pages, we strive to keep our standards at Yahweh Yoga above reproach.

The model for our photography is Courtney Kutta, my amazing daughter and co-founder of Yahweh Yoga. All the posture instructions were also written by her. Courtney is an inspired teacher who loves the Lord with all of her heart. Our heartfelt prayer is that you enjoy the health that comes through Christ-centered self-care for your body and soul.

Yours in Christ,

DeAnna Smothers, E-RYT, CCYT
Co-Founder & CEO
Yahweh Yoga, LLC
December 2007, Phoenix

A Prayer for Beginning

Lord, we're tired.

We're hungry and thirsty but we don't know what for.

>Our bodies hurt.

>Our hearts ache.

We want to enter a spacious place where we can

>move freely,

>breathe deeply,

>be at ease in our own skin.

We want to come to You and lay our burdens down.

>Teach us your unforced rhythms of grace.

>Teach us how to live in a way that is easy and light.

>Teach us your ways.

Restore us, O God, make your face shine upon us, that we may be saved.

>Refresh our tired bodies, restore our tired souls.

>Set our feet in your spacious place.

Lead us to green pastures.

>Lead us in the way everlasting.

>Lead us into your presence.

Into Your presence we come.

He brought me out into
a spacious place;
he rescued me because
he delighted in me.
PSALM 18:19

The LORD is my shepherd,
I shall not be in want.
He makes me lie down
in green pastures,
He leads me beside quiet waters,
He restores my soul.
PSALM 23:1-3

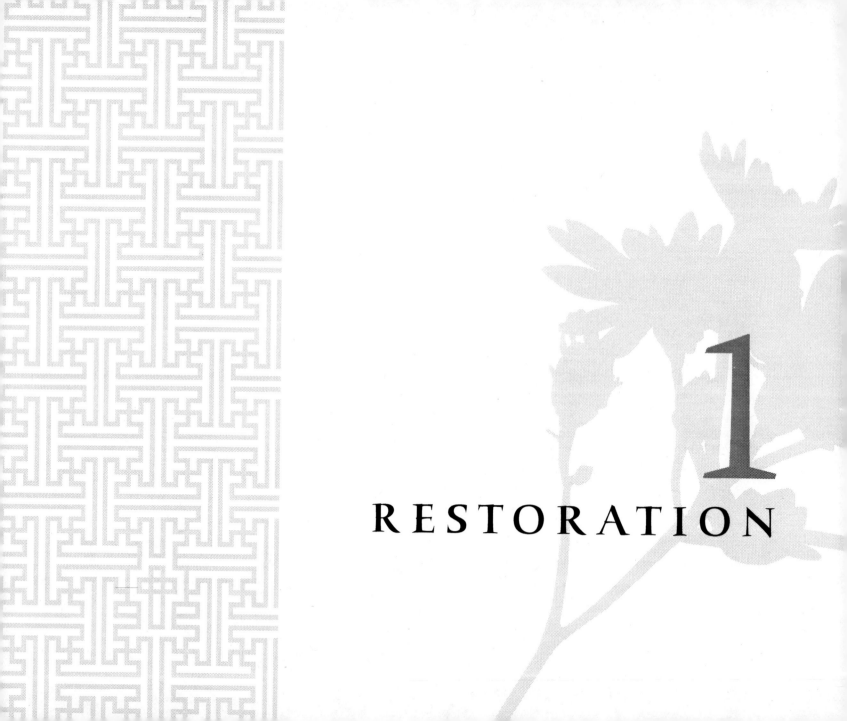

RESTORATION

1

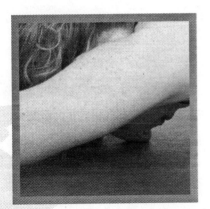 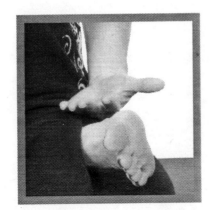 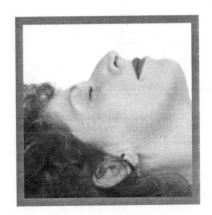

Restore us, O God.
PSALM 80:3

CHAPTER ONE

Tired Bodies & Tired Souls

"ALTHOUGH WE NEVER anticipate a change in cabin pressure, should one occur, four oxygen masks will fall from the compartment above. Place the mask over your nose and mouth and breathe normally. If you are traveling with small children please secure your own mask first and then assist the child. Continue wearing the mask until otherwise notified by a uniformed crewmember. Finally sit back, relax, and enjoy your flight!"

Restore us, O God; make your face shine upon us, that we may be saved.
PSALM 80:3

I'll refresh tired bodies, I'll restore tired souls.
JEREMIAH 31:25 THE MESSAGE

"Are you clear on the safety instructions?" asked the flight attendant as she paused at my seat.

"Yes," I said and smiled. "We've been flying with our children since they were babies. We're all familiar with the rules." Or so I thought.

"Hey, that's not right," my son said accusingly, after the attendant moved on. "Parents are supposed to look after kids first."

"Mom, why should grownups get the oxygen before kids?" my daughter asked anxiously. "Will there be enough for us?"

"Adults need to put on their mask first so they can breathe the oxygen and be able to help the kids," I explained. "I am much bigger than you and if I pass out you won't be able to help me and I, for sure, won't be able to help you then. And, yes, there is enough oxygen for everyone." They relaxed as I assured them it was in their best interest for mom and dad to be first this time.

As we settled into our flight it occurred to me that these instructions would be helpful for life in general. Pressurized life changes happen to us all the time but no automatic oxygen masks fall down in front of us. So often we look into the eyes of those depending on us (a child, spouse, parent, boss, neighbor or the PTO or church committee) and we feel the pressure starting to squeeze the life out of us. We know we are starting to run out of air and desperately need to find an oxygen mask. But we don't. We muddle on, asthmatic and wheezing in our feeble efforts to meet everyone's needs.

Many of us get caught in this cycle of personal neglect that helps no one. We are pulled in a hundred different directions by competing demands for our time and attention. We feel exhausted, stressed and fragmented. Opportunities and obligations overwhelm us and we struggle to make appropriate choices. Our bodies and our souls ache as we grope for rhythm and direction. Longing for someone to give us permission to look after ourselves —to secure our own mask first —we crave restoration.

Restoration

In the Bible we see so many beautiful images and promises of God's restoration. The Psalmist speaks of the Lord, our shepherd, restoring our soul. God tells us of his longing and plans to restore his people, Israel. Jeremiah writes, "But I will restore you to health and heal your wounds, declares the Lord"(Jeremiah 30:17).

Jesus' ministry on earth included restoration. He healed the sick and wounded and restored their health. He mended the brokenhearted and restored their peace. He forgave sinners, restoring their relationships with God. Jesus still does that today. He cares deeply about each one of us and in him we can find the true refreshment we crave for our bodies and souls. Jesus extends this invitation to us:

> Come to me, all you who are weary and burdened, and I will give you rest. Take my yoke upon you and learn from me, for I am gentle and humble in heart, and you will find rest for your souls. For my yoke is easy and my burden is light. (Matthew 11:28)

Christian Yoga: Restoration for Body and Soul offers an invitation to come and lay down your burdens, to take off the yoke of the world and pick up Christ's easy yoke instead. Within these pages we examine what it means to look after ourselves and why it is so hard to do. Christian yoga is presented as an ideal means of self-care and we take a close look at the questions and concerns about it. We consider practical needs of both body and soul and how we can meet those needs. The last section includes detailed and illustrated instructions for yoga postures to help you in your pursuit of physical health and strength. Throughout we develop and maintain a clear purpose and vision for our self-care: we care for ourselves in order to love and serve God and others better.

We want to discover how to secure our oxygen masks so we can breathe freely even when life surprises us. It is possible! We need not continue wheezing and gasping for air under the crushing pressures of life. We can respond to Christ's invitation and step into a place where we breathe deeply and feel renewed. Let's learn together how to pursue appropriate self-care and find restoration for our body and soul, keeping in mind God's wonderful promise to refresh our tired bodies and restore our tired souls.

CHAPTER TWO
Self-care

IN *THE ART OF TRAVEL*, Alain de Botton describes for us a beautiful morning on a beach in Barbados. He has left the cold English winter for the warm sands of a Caribbean paradise. Surprisingly, he finds his ability to appreciate the idyllic scene in front of him marred by

> a sore throat I had developed during the flight, worry over not having informed a colleague that I would be away, a pressure across both temples and a rising need to visit the bathroom. A momentous but until then overlooked fact was making itself apparent: *I had inadvertently brought myself with me to the island.*[1]

No matter how we might try or where we might fly we can't escape the *self* or ignore its needs and anxieties. We accompany ourselves where ever we go.

"Self" is a very popular word today. With no end of self-help books and seminars, we are encouraged to seek self-actualization and try to get in touch with the true self or the deep self. We desire to be self-sufficient and self-assured. We worry about our self-worth and self-esteem. We admire self-sacrifice and self-control and struggle to be more self-disciplined. We may not care too much for the self-absorbed or self-centered yet we like the self-confident. We're self-employed, self-appointed, self-conscious, self-deprecating, self-congratulatory and self-contained. We are bombarded with The Self. Yet we struggle to find a clear definition of balanced and appropriate self-care.

Love the Lord your God with all your heart and with all your soul and with all your strength and with all your mind; and love your neighbor as yourself.
LUKE 10:27

My purpose is to love God completely, love self correctly, and love others compassionately.
KENNETH BOA

When we read the beautiful promise in Jeremiah 31 in *The Message* that God will "refresh tired bodies and restore tired souls" we discover that it is surrounded by many imperatives: *return, go back, resume, repent, enjoy, dance, be happy, come, let's go to meet our God.* God waits and longs for us to come to him. "O Ephraim is my dear, dear son, my child in whom I take pleasure! Every time I mention his name, my heart bursts with longing for him! Everything in me cries out for him. Softly and tenderly I wait for him"(v.20). Softly and tenderly, God is waiting for you too.

God calls us to *come* to him and be ready participants in the process of renewal. Caring for ourselves requires that we be actively involved, not passively waiting for God to zap us with renewed energy and health. Leading up to God's promise of restoration, we find instructions to *mark our trip home, get a good map, study the road conditions* and *come back, come back* (v. 21-22). We thrive or flounder depending on how much responsibility we take for our own well-being.

When we take those first steps on the road to accepting God's invitation to come find rest, refreshment and restoration, he meets us there. Caring for ourselves starts with acknowledging that God is the source of our life and our only hope for restoration. Then we accept the invitation to step into the process of restoration, to come to him. Self-care also expresses good stewardship of God's gracious gifts. Our life is a gift. We thank him for this gift by caring for the needs of our bodies and souls.

Body and Soul

It is a mystery how our bodies, hearts, minds, spirits and souls come together to form the "self". We may not understand how that works but we can't ignore the different facets of the self. Balanced self-care recognizes that we all have real physical, emotional, mental and spiritual needs.

I can devote lots of time and energy to physical exercise and achieve a high level of fitness. If I neglect my soul in the process I may be able to run a marathon but I risk being uptight, anxious and maybe even irritable. In the same way, I can devote lots of time and energy to the needs of my soul and aim to perfectly bear all the fruit of the spirit. I may never yell at my kids but I also may not be able to run and play with them if my body is falling apart because of neglect. I don't think I like either of these options. Care for just the body or for just the soul creates imbalance. We don't have to compromise one for the other, however. Instead, we can find ideal self-care practices that integrate and address the needs of body and soul together, in balance.

Finding Balance Between Self-Neglect and Self-Worship

When we approach the idea of self-care we want to avoid another area of imbalance: the pitfalls of self-neglect and self-worship. The challenge is to love ourselves appropriately.

I doubt many of us wake up and say, "Hey, I am going to neglect myself today!" Sad cases of self-abuse do exist, but more often self-neglect creeps up on us in the midst of greater competing demands for our attention. We don't have the time or energy to address our personal needs and they fall to the bottom of the to-do list. Suddenly we feel cranky and we're carrying an extra twenty pounds. Our friends and family start talking about nominating us for *What Not to Wear*. Our children wonder what happened to our "happy-face" and our "nice words." We all know this doesn't really happen suddenly. Self-neglect often reflects a poor assessment of our self-worth. Failing to properly look after ourselves can also be an indicator of more serious conditions like depression, anxiety, stress or burnout.

Self-neglect is different than self-sacrifice. Self-sacrifice knowingly sets aside your own valid needs for a time, in order to meet others' needs. In contrast, self-neglect is generally unintentional or a sign that you have decided (consciously or not) that your needs are not valid in the first place. Self-sacrifice and self-denial are legitimate, necessary and good choices that we make in life. Jesus said that "whoever tries to keep his life will lose it and whoever loses his life will preserve it."[2] He also told his disciples, "If anyone wants to be first, he must be the very last, and the servant of all."[3] When we follow Jesus, we embrace the privileges of service and sacrifice. We will be so much better able to make these choices of sacrifice and to welcome opportunities for service when we start from a position of self-care rather than neglect.

When we end the cycle of self-neglect and instead, start caring for ourselves, we make some pretty powerful assumptions about who we are. We declare that we are worth caring for. This is a truth proclaimed throughout the Bible. Genesis tells us that God made us in his image and pronounced his creation good. The Psalmist marvels at how we are each fearfully and wonderfully made and that God knows each of our days before one of them is yet to be. God is intimately acquainted and concerned with us and loves us so much that he sent his son to die to reconcile us with himself. Surely, if God cares for us that much then we are worth caring for ourselves.

We also declare that self-care is a good thing to do. Again, this assumption is consistent with Scripture. Consider all the warnings in Proverbs against sloth, gluttony and foolishness. Romans exhorts us not to offer our bodies as instruments of unrighteousness and Galatians extols the fruit of the spirit: love, joy, peace, patience, kindness, goodness, faithfulness, gentleness and self-control. Paul reminds us in 1 Corinthians 6:19-20 that our "body is a temple of the Holy Spirit, who is in you; whom you have received from God. You are not your own; you were bought at a price. Therefore, honor God with your body." Respect the gift God has given you and the investment he has made in you.

When we choose to reverse trends of self-neglect and care for our bodies and our souls, we honor God.

At the opposite end of the spectrum from self-neglect lies self-worship. Where self-neglect comes from sliding priorities and a lack of self-worth, self-worship declares that I am the only priority and my needs are the only ones that shall be met. Self-worship showcases just as many unhealthy habits as self-neglect. When we worship ourselves our appearance may become the most important thing. Our self-worth gets wrapped up in whether others find us attractive or not. We constantly evaluate our relationships and our engagements against whether *our* needs are satisfied. If not, we feel free to walk away from those commitments and relationships. Paul warned Timothy that in the last days "people will be *lovers of themselves*, lovers of money, boastful, proud, abusive, disobedient to their parents, ungrateful, unholy, without love, unforgiving, slanderous, without self-control, brutal, not lovers of the good, treacherous, rash, conceited, lovers of pleasure rather than lovers of God"(1 Timothy 3:2-3, emphasis added).

Lovers of themselves... In this age of YouTube, reality TV and the extreme makeover, you need not look far for spectacular displays of this kind of narcissism. I am amazed by the poor behavior showcased in so many of these shows. I don't know how to reconcile the apparently low standards for conduct with the unrealistically high standards for appearance in the makeover shows. *You don't like the way God made you? Let's change you into somebody you can really love.* Every time I open my email inbox right now, a banner ad promises me I can "Get the body of a hottie" if I buy their nutritional supplements. Other ads offer reconstructive surgery or miracle injections. We can erase all evidence of child bearing, unhealthy habits and disappointing genes. It really is tempting, I know! But when we stake our happiness on looking good enough, we will always be disappointed.

We avoid the trap of self-worship by aiming higher than the desires to conform to the unrealistic images and expectations laid on us by the world; by aiming higher than the "new and improved self." Our ability to live in balance and love ourselves correctly without falling into self-neglect or self-worship hinges on our focus and motivation. In our pursuit of balanced self-care what we really want is to be transformed from the inside out. We don't want to be merely lovers of ourselves. We want to be lovers of God and people.

Loving God First and Loving Others: Ordering Principles for Self-Care

One day a young man called out to Jesus, "Lord, what is the most important commandment?"

"The most important one," answered Jesus, "is this: 'Hear, O Israel, the Lord our God, the Lord is one. Love the Lord your God with all your heart and with all your soul and with all your mind and with all your strength.' The second is this: 'Love your neighbor as yourself.' There is no commandment greater than these" (Mark 12:28-33).

The focus and motivation for our self-care lies in Jesus' answer to this essential question of humanity. *Why are we here?* We are here to love God with our whole being, with everything we've got, and to love others as we love ourselves. Bradley Holt, author of *Thirsty for God*, helps us understand what that means.

> The Bible generally views a person as a unity of body, soul, mind, heart and spirit. It does not separate these elements the way some philosophers have. Thus the self in the Bible is the whole person, including the body, soul, intellect, will, emotions, conscious and unconscious, and social and private, whatever distinctions have been made. It is this whole self that is called upon to love, serve and praise God. [4]

When we draw these lines around the different parts of ourselves we tend to draw similar boundaries around our relationships and activities. So our tendency may be to think of our relationship with God as something that only happens at certain times or in certain ways. Instead, when we love, serve and praise God with the whole self those boundaries are blurred and we find new ways of experiencing and expressing our relationship with him. Every part of our life, even the ordinary every-day parts, becomes an opportunity to live a life of worship. There is a place in your relationship with God for your self-care. In fact, it is only in this relationship that we find our true self-worth and the motivation and direction for our self-care that we need.

Loving Others As You Love Yourself

The second greatest commandment flows from this primary relationship. When we love God and are loved by him, we begin to share his heart and love for our neighbor. Why do we look after ourselves? Caring for ourselves is really not about us. It's about others. Here is the defining paradox of Christian self-care that sets it apart from other self-care systems: ultimately it does not focus on the self. Our focus is outward, centered on God and oriented toward service. We are called to be servants and to love and glorify God with every aspect of our being. We are his workmanship, created in Christ Jesus to do good works, which he has already prepared for us to do[5]. Neglected bodies and souls distract and interfere with our primary purpose.* Likewise, self-absorption prevents us from stepping into those good works and living the life of a servant.

---

* Let me be careful to point out that many of us suffer physical pain and conditions over which we have no control and no ability to modify. In this situation I believe our calling is to participate as far as we are able to in the pursuit of as much health as we can attain. The primary concern of this book is to identify those areas that we may be neglecting and where we have the power to make choices for change. For example, a paraplegic can't reverse her paralysis if she just works up enough willpower. But she does have the power to make choices of how to best live with that condition and pursue health with the means available to her.

God sets the standard for how we are to love others—*as we love ourselves*. Some have taken this standard and have misapplied it to justify a rather robust self-love that in practice does not leave room for others. Others have made a pre-requisite of self-love—we must have sufficiently loved ourselves *before* we start to love and care for others. *As yourself* means, love others with the same diligence and care that you apply to your own needs and do this *as* you are meeting your own needs.

In our quest to walk the middle way between self-neglect and self-worship I think we err on the side of neglect more often. We tend to set a higher standard than God's for how we look after others' needs in contrast to how we look after ourselves. I know as a wife and mom I wrestle with finding and maintaining the balance I need. How do I juggle my responsibilities to God, my self and others? I race and struggle to meet everyone else's demands and needs, depleting my resources and running on empty. I feel guilty for not loving God with everything I've got and wonder if I love others enough, forgetting that looking after myself is a good thing to do. I'm sure you do too. We get worn out, rung out and fed up. We know we need to look after ourselves but knowledge and agreement don't seem to be enough to make it happen. We stumble up against some common roadblocks. Be encouraged! With our new perspective and right motivation for our self-care we can overcome these challenges to getting it done.

Overcoming Obstacles

Why is it so hard to make self-care a priority? I think it's because you and I are usually trying to choose among equally good and legitimate demands for our time. Do I volunteer in my child's classroom or do I go to yoga class while I am free during school hours? Do you visit your sick friend with a meal, go grocery shopping or find some quiet time for yourself? These are challenging choices but we can set priorities that work for us if we keep a few things in mind.

1. First, let's remember our new perspective and motivation for our self-care. We are worth caring for. We honor God when we look after ourselves. Our motivation is to be better able to love and serve God and others. Simply put, everything else on our to-do list will be done better when we pay attention to our needs. So self-care deserves a priority spot on the list.

2. It's okay to say no! Maybe you need to hear that again. Read it aloud. **It's okay to say no**. Sometimes we have to say no to good things and even things that we really want to do because we can't do it all. We can't *be* it all either. I want to be it all. Don't you? I've learned the hard way that saying yes to every good opportunity is ultimately more painful than the regret of turning things down. If you struggle with this it may be helpful to

remember that when you say no you create an opportunity for someone else to say yes. (Now, isn't that generous of you?)

3. We can negotiate our choices. Not everything is an either/or proposition. With some creativity and planning we can create opportunities for self-care that we may have not recognized before. Look for where you might combine some tasks with your self-care goals. Maybe you can walk to and from school when you volunteer in the classroom. Discuss with your spouse how you can work together to share responsibilities and free each other up to exercise body and soul. Start small: find one time a week to go to a Christian yoga class and buy a DVD to help you practice at home.

4. Keep it simple! David Allen is one of the leading business and time management gurus of the moment. His million dollar mantra? *Getting things done*™. Don't you wish you had trademarked that one? At the end of the day we need to put one foot in front of the other and just get it done. Have that necessary discussion with your spouse, your co-workers or your children, set boundaries, rearrange schedules, write inspirational post-it notes to yourself—whatever it takes. In the immortal words of Nike, "Just Do It!"

5. Finally, and really this should be first, take your lists and everything that is clamoring for your attention and lay it before God. He is our ultimate priority setter. Time with God

helps us gain the heavenly perspective we need and is a fundamental part of our self-care. Ask him to guide you in managing your responsibilities and goals.

Now that we have a new perspective on balanced self-care it helps to have a way to do it. You may already be familiar with the benefits of regularly practicing yoga but feel uneasy about it as a Christian. We want to show you how Christian yoga offers a unique God-honoring means of self-care that addresses the needs of body and soul in one practice. One of my challenges in looking after my self is finding enough time for both physical exercise and quiet time with God. I started attending Christian yoga classes because I desperately needed to do something for my back and arthritis. My body was falling apart and I was way too young for that to happen. I got excited about Christian yoga because my soul was nourished at the same time. Instead of feeling rushed and anxious about getting in both exercise and quiet time I left yoga class ready to tackle the rest of my day, renewed in my energy and spirit through the exercise, worship, meditation and self-examination. I went to class to fix my body and discovered how starved my soul was for uninterrupted time with God.

Many share a story like mine. On the door to our studio are these words: *An Oasis for Self-Care.* The classes and community at Yahweh Yoga have truly been an oasis for many men and women seeking restoration of their bodies and their souls. Some of their stories are in this book. We have had the privilege of ministering to people suffering through grief,

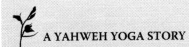

A YAHWEH YOGA STORY

As a Christian yoga teacher I see so much healing. I have seen people over time become quiet before the Lord and watched Him bring peace, joy and balance to their lives.

Not that the dramas of life go away. But we can feel calmer, healing both mind, body and spirit. Many of my students have been restored through the wonderful practice of Christian Yoga and it is a joy to see.

—Janet

divorce, cancer and other stressful experiences. It is not unusual for teachers and class members to gather around and pray for one of our hurting students at the end of class. What a joy it is to observe God bringing healing and restoration and to be given the privilege of teaching his children basic principles of self-care. You too can use the principles of Christian yoga, which we will examine next, for a balanced approach to wellness and wholeness that is motivated by love for God and others.

So, what is Christian yoga? Isn't that an oxymoron? Can Christians really practice yoga and still be Christians? Let's investigate this together. Put on your thinking caps and strap in. We're about to take a whirlwind tour of history, comparative religions, philosophy and the Bible in our quest to address these concerns.

---

[1] Alain de Botton, *The Art of Travel*, (New York, Vintage International, 2004) p.19, emphasis added.
[2] Luke 17:33
[3] Mark 9:35
[4] Bradley Holt, *Thirsty for God: A Brief History of Christian Spirituality*, (Minneapolis: Fortress Press, 2005), p. 27.
[5] Ephesians 2:10

CHAPTER THREE

What is Yoga?

I HAVE STRUGGLED with chronic back pain for most of my life. As I entered my thirties I started to exhibit symptoms of arthritis and was very discouraged. A number of friends and doctors recommended yoga. I knew yoga had the potential to help me find relief but I was uncertain about it. I wasn't sure if it was an appropriate practice for Christians but everything I read about yoga seemed to promise exactly what I needed. "I wish there was something like Christian yoga," I whined to my husband on many occasions. Apparently God listens to whining. Within months of expressing that desire (many times) I was introduced to the women who founded Yahweh Yoga, DeAnna Smothers and Courtney Kutta. As I experienced the classes and researched the history and origins of yoga I became excited. I could see the potential for a beautiful practice of body and soul that would help Christians in their desire to be healthy and growing, both physically and spiritually.

Many Christians have shared my experience and my uncertainty. Maybe you too have wished that you could enjoy the benefits of yoga but have been uncertain about whether you could freely do that as a follower of Christ. These are legitimate concerns and we need to be careful in evaluating yoga as a practice for Christians. We need to exercise great discernment in recognizing what is honoring to God and what is not. There are a lot of big ideas to consider here but let's take a look together at how we can understand and answer the questions about Christian yoga.

Test everything. Hold on to the good.
Avoid every kind of evil.
1 THESSALONIANS 5:21-22

For the LORD gives wisdom,
and from his mouth come knowledge
and understanding.
PROVERBS 2:6

Hatha Yoga

Very little is known about the origins of the practice of yoga. The earliest written record of yoga is in the Vedantic scriptures dating back about 1500 years. However, archaeological finds in the Indus valley show depictions of yoga postures dating back 3000 to 5000 BC. It is reasonable to conclude that the practice of yoga postures predates the development of today's major world religions. Indeed, it is overwhelmingly stated throughout yoga literature that yoga is not a religion. These assertions are made by those of Hindu, Buddhist, Christian and other faiths. Rather, yoga is a discipline that may be practiced within or without the context of any faith.

What is recognized generally as yoga in our society today is actually one branch of yoga philosophy called hatha yoga. When we speak of yoga in this book we refer specifically to the practice of hatha yoga. Hatha yoga stresses wellness of the body and soul through the use of postures and purposeful breathing, self examination and meditation. A leading hatha yoga cardiac therapist, Nirmala Heriza, gives us this definition of yoga: "Yoga is a complete science or synthesis of practices—the poses (asanas), meditation, self analysis, nutrition, self awareness—that when combined influence and inform not just our physical body but also our mental, emotional and spiritual health."[1]

This definition comes pretty close to our ideal for self-care: practices that integrate the needs of body and soul together in balance. Christian yoga seeks to employ the healthy and beneficial practices of hatha yoga as a support to the pursuit of physical health and spiritual growth. Christian yoga assumes that God is the origin of all truth and beauty and that things that are true can be redeemed and consecrated for His glory. Paul warned Timothy against people who made up rules that God never intended, like forbidding marriage or certain foods. He tells Timothy that instead "everything God created is good, and nothing is to be rejected if it is received with thanksgiving, because it is consecrated by the word of God and prayer" (1 Timothy 4:4-5).

I think that similarly we can thank God for how he created our bodies and enjoy physical movement, like yoga, that brings health to our bodies. God's creation reveals truth about him and likewise our bodies are a revelation of his wisdom as the Ultimate Designer. Our bodies work best in the way he designed them to work and practices that support the healthy function of our bodies are ultimately from Him.

The word *yoga* comes from the Sanskrit *yug* which can be translated as "to harmonize", "to bring together" or "to harness or yoke". As Christians we can apply this image of yoking in a couple of ways. First, we can understand it as the idea of desiring wholeness or unity in our person of the physical, spiritual, mental and emotional aspects of our being. We seek to yoke together all these parts to be able to move forward with purpose just as a farmer yokes his oxen together to move the plow in one direction. We pursue an integrated focused life instead of a fragmented life.

We can also apply the picture of being yoked to pursuing harmony or communion with God, bringing our lives in line with Him. We seek to be yoked in relationship with God and by God. Jesus uses this image or metaphor when he invites us to take off the world's harness and take on his yoke instead:

> Come to me, all you who are weary and burdened, and I will give you rest. Take my *yoke* upon you and learn from me, for I am gentle and humble in heart, and you will find rest for your souls. For my *yoke* is easy and my burden is light (Matthew 11:28, emphasis added).

There is a beautiful parallel between the picture Jesus draws for us here and the image of yoking in Christian yoga. When we practice Christian yoga we can keep this picture in our minds and imagine surrendering our fragmented and distracted lives to his lordship, to be transformed and conformed to his image and redirected under his yoke of grace and mercy. This is one way we consecrate the practice of Christian yoga.

How is Christian yoga different?

While it is noteworthy that the practice of yoga predates the development of today's world religions and that it does not claim to be a religion itself, that is not sufficient alone as a basis for the practice of *Christian* yoga. It was within the context of eastern pantheistic and monistic[2] religions that yoga was developed and codified. Therefore most of the different types and expressions of yoga philosophy are anchored in a belief system that does **not** acknowledge God as the one true God, creator of heaven and earth and creator of man, nor acknowledges Christ as the Way, the Truth and the Life and the only path of salvation or means of reconciliation with God. So we need to be discerning about what we incorporate from eastern yoga traditions in the practice of Christian yoga.

In our western society, most people recognize yoga as a physical practice, sometimes with a benign spiritual emphasis added. You can easily find yoga classes with no spiritual component but you can also find yoga that is heavily spiritual and even cultic. The spiritual aspects of yoga most commonly expressed in our western culture are generally an amalgam of Hindu, Buddhist and New Age beliefs and practices. While often sincere, it is usually a murky mix of spiritual practices with blurred boundaries between the philosophical origins and ideas.

Subtleties of language and questionable ideas can easily creep into a yoga practice if we are not careful to recognize them and their origin. This is where a Christian must apply diligence and discernment. There is nothing inherently spiritual (good or evil) about a leg bend or downward dog – it is the ideas and objectives that attach themselves to the physical practice that must be carefully considered.

delayed. You feel an immense difference in mind and body as soon as class is over as well as increased strength, stamina, and stability over time. Yahweh Yoga has become a crucial ingredient in my health. I highly recommend it for anyone.

—Patty

For example, in Hindu yoga, some methods of breath control seek to liberate the soul from the constraints of the body which is illusion and promote transcendence to another spiritual plane. That is an idea that is fundamentally incompatible with the Christian worldview of humanity, the material and spiritual worlds and God. Understanding our worldview in contrast with other worldviews will help us to recognize and discern these ideas that may lead us away from truth. As Christians, our worldview—our assumptions about who we are, who God is and the world we live in—informs our practice of yoga and changes the nature of what we do.

Let's take a look at some of the key ideas in these worldviews and compare them to a biblical worldview. A vast divide exists between western thought, which embraces reason, and eastern thought, which generally rejects any usefulness of reason. So it is challenging to examine these differences but we can do it. We will consider the concept of the self and it's relationship to the physical world and divinity in the primary worldviews represented in Hinduism and Buddhism, the two religious systems that have influenced yoga the most and that brought yoga to the western world.

The Self, the World and God in Hinduism

Hinduism is not a religion so much as a collection of many belief systems with multiple expressions and gods. There are some core philosophies and beliefs however. For the

Hindu, the self or *atman*, is an uncreated soul that exists eternally and must be recycled through many lives (*samsara*). The self is indistinct from the universal soul, or Supreme Being which is everywhere and in everything. This is pantheism: God or the Supreme Being is all and is in all.

Reincarnation can even send the soul into forms other than human life, such as animals, plants or even objects. Through one's actions, *karma* is collected, either positive or negative, and one's karma determines the next reincarnation. Suffering is earned and is proportionate to a person's karma. Salvation, or escape from the endless cycle of rebirth, comes through collecting enough karma to ascend the ladder of life and be reincarnated as progressively higher beings. The goal is for atman to be rejoined with Brahman, the universal soul or Ultimate Reality.

A key saying in Hinduism is, "Atman is Brahman." In other words there is no essential difference between man or man's soul and the divine. The goal of reunion of atman with Brahman is like a cup of water being poured into a lake. The water in the cup is in essence and nature identical to the lake—it is kept from the lake by the constraints of the cup. Once the water is returned to the lake it ceases to be separate or distinguishable in any way. Likewise, the soul dissolves into the impersonal Ultimate Reality and ceases to be. For the Hindu, atman is kept from Brahman by the constraints of the body or life in the natural world which is understood to be illusory or unreal (*maya*). Therefore the material world and its comforts and its suffering are not real. Release from this illusion and from the wheel of life is called *moksha*.

There is some irony here. A system of belief that denies material reality and denies that physical suffering is real (even though it is earned or deserved) has been a primary contributor to the development of hatha yoga, a practice of health that is objectively and eminently beneficial for the physical body and for the relief of physical pain and suffering.

The Self, the World and God in Buddhism

Gautama Buddha became disillusioned with trying to follow the ways of Hinduism to achieve personal freedom and developed his own philosophy of life instead. While the Hindu believes there is no real physical body, the Buddhist believes there is no real or enduring self or soul. What is misconceived of as the self is merely an aggregate of constantly changing and mutating factors and therefore impermanent and unreal. Clinging to the false notion of a real self or soul only leads to unhappiness or suffering. Since Buddhists believe in reincarnation this raises a problem: if there is no enduring self, what then is reincarnated? This paradox of the non-soul and reincarnation has occupied much of Buddhist philosophy and immense effort is employed to fully grasp the concept of the non-self.

Since Buddhism evolved out of Hinduism, it has retained some Hindu principles but has rejected others. Buddha did not accept that the present world and life in it was unreal or illusion (*maya*). Instead he affirmed the reality of the material world and life in it which is marked by real suffering. In Buddhism the source of suffering is attachment to and desire for the world and life. The only way to cease suffering is to escape the endless wheel of life (of the non-self) into nirvana. One escapes the wheel through self-effort toward enlightenment or correctly realizing one's non-existence. Nirvana means "to cease" or "to extinguish". Buddhists will deny that their system is nihilistic, but when you follow the logical path of Buddhist principles, nihilism is the end result.

Buddhism generally rejects that there is a divine being or supreme being. There are many different branches of Buddhism with differences in philosophies, however, and in these various expressions you will find worship of divinities, idols and/or ancestors. The Hindu Brahmin priests declared Buddha an incarnation of their god Vishnu but Buddha never claimed divinity himself.

In summary, our quick survey of the two religious systems that have most influenced and used yoga reveals worldviews that differ greatly from the Christian worldview. The self or soul is either a non-existent fiction that we must strive to free ourselves from, or an uncreated and eternal essence indistinct from the Supreme Being. The material world is fiction or the source of our suffering—either way it must be escaped. Suffering is caused by attachment to illusions or to the material world or by insufficient karma and good works. God is either non-existent or everywhere and in everything, one in essence with man and impersonal.

The Self, the World and God in the Christian Worldview

In contrast, the biblical worldview asserts that we are made by God in his image and that his creation is good. Psalm 139 tells us that God created our "inmost being" and that we are "fearfully and wonderfully made." Colossians 1:16 says that "all things are created by him and for him." We are his workmanship, body and soul, and we are intended for relationship with him. Sin entered the perfect world through Adam and corrupted the world and separated man from God but he offers us reconciliation through Christ's saving work on the cross. If we trust in him we have the hope of eternal life. God is completely other than us, distinct from his creation but intimately involved with it as Creator, Redeemer and Sustainer. The self is real (both in body and in soul), the world is real, both are good and both are not God.

Therefore, when we as Christians practice yoga as a discipline of health for body and soul, our assumptions about our bodies and souls create a unique paradigm for our practice. We are not meditating to fully grasp the concept of the unreal world or the non-existence of self. We are not controlling our breath in order to release our inner self from our illusory body to transcend to another, more real, spiritual plane. We are not practicing a physical asceticism in order to more deeply comprehend the fictional nature of our body. We are not seeking union or yoking with Ultimate reality. We don't hope for nirvana or for our souls to be extinguished or re-assimilated.

Instead, we meditate on God and his Word because he has instructed us to. We breathe deeply and purposefully because that is the way God in his wisdom designed our bodies to function. We honor God by caring for our bodies which are a real and good creation of God. We move our bodies in ways that support the functions of his miraculous design. Our soul does not seek release or transcendence or union—we seek communion with our Maker in the personal relationship he made us for. And when our brief journey this side of heaven is finished, our hope is eternal life with God.

There is a difference between a theory and practice or between a theology and a method. For example, prayer is common to all religions and even people who profess no faith will admit to praying. Prayer is a method. It is our theology and our faith that employs prayer, defines our prayers as uniquely Christian, and gives meaning and substance to our prayers. But a Buddhist or a Hindu will also pray, so likewise, their theology makes their prayers different than ours.

We've just examined some of the different theories and theologies that use yoga as a *method*. In the same way as prayer, yoga is a method or means that we can employ in our pursuit of physical health and our spiritual formation, our being transformed and conformed to the image of Christ. But when we use yoga as a method it is of essence entirely different than yoga used as a method by a Buddhist, Hindu or New Age disciple. Christian yoga is defined by our theology, never the other way around.

Avoiding Syncretism—Centered on Christ, Anchored in Scripture

Our challenge as Christians is not to figure out how our life in Christ can be incorporated into or made compatible with yoga. This would be syncretism which is the mixing and fusing of different systems of belief. Syncretism is never advocated in the Bible. Repeatedly in Scripture, God tells us he is the one TRUE God and that we shall have no other gods before him. Throughout the Old Testament Israel was told to be holy, set apart, not to intermarry with other faiths, not to worship other gods. Similarly, we want to consecrate our Christian yoga practice, not mix it in with other faiths. Our practice of yoga must always be subordinate to our life in Christ and subject to scrutiny against the truth in the Scripture.

As Christians we declare that there is only one way to God and that is through Christ—the Truth, the Way and the Life. Two errors that we need to guard against in practicing Christian yoga are:

- Viewing Christ as just another way to salvation that is worthy of consideration, or merely viewing him as a better way.

- Putting a veneer of Christ on top of practices that deny him. We might do this with surface signs of Christianity in our language or our environment while leaving the substance unchanged.

We guard against syncretism by keeping Christ at the center of Christian yoga and anchoring our practice in Scripture, exercising wisdom and discernment. Our challenge as followers of Christ is to examine yoga carefully and identify:

- The beneficial physical (non-spiritual) elements.

- The beneficial spiritual practices (meditation, body expression of worship, self examination) that are compatible with Christian spirituality.

- The philosophies and practices that are incompatible with Christ and our life in Him.

In using yoga as a self-care practice, we also want to evaluate it against our standards for self-care. Does this help me love God with all my heart, soul, mind and strength? Does this help me love people? Am I being motivated to love God and others or am I being led in self-centeredness?

Addressing Additional Concerns

Does performing yoga postures and flows result in the Christian inadvertently worshiping Hindu Deities or engaging unwittingly in occult practices?

Imagine this scene with me: Garlic and the scent of warm bread in the brick ovens suffuse the air. Red-checked table cloths cover the closely packed dinner tables and the trattoria resonates with the laughter and chatter of satisfied diners. A bottle of fine chianti and a crusty loaf rest on most tables. Suddenly, the heavens open and a firestorm engulfs the restaurant, incinerating all the patrons within—*for inadvertently partaking of communion in an unworthy manner.*

Absurd? Of course it is. Commonsense tells us that it is the intention and heart of the participants that invest a ritual or symbolic practice with meaning, not the mere elements. The specific postures that seem to raise this question about yoga the most are those included in the flow known as the Sun Salutation.

The Sun Salutation is traditionally performed early in the morning upon rising and is a simple greeting of the day. The postures include lifting your arms and face upward and forward bends. Does everyone who raises their face and arms to the heavens participate in sun worship? No. We lift our hands to worship God and we praise him for his glorious creation and the precious gift of a new day, following the examples of God's people in his word. *This is the day the Lord has made. Let us rejoice and be glad in it! Your compassions are new every morning. Great is your faithfulness. We revere your name; for us the sun of righteousness will rise with healing in its wings.*[3]

By stretching our arms toward heaven or leaning over in a forward bend we won't be participating in a form of Hindu worship or occult ritual unknowingly, anymore than someone who makes the sign of the cross invokes a magical blessing, or anyone who enjoys a glass of wine and bread with their dinner unknowingly partakes of communion. Tilden Edwards has stated that, "What makes a particular practice Christian is not its source, but its intent. If our intent in assuming a particular bodily practice is to deepen our awareness in Christ, then it is Christian. If this is not our intent in any spiritual practice, then even the reading of Scripture loses its Christian authenticity."[4]

It is also interesting to note that you find many of the same postures as yoga in physical therapy, Pilates and old-fashioned calisthenics. If these body movements are exclusively Hindu expressions of worship, then the Hindu deities are getting a lot of extra devotion in therapy clinics and fitness centers throughout the world.

Intention and purpose are key. However, we must also be diligent in exercising wisdom and discernment to evaluate the practices we are going to assume. We all know the old proverb, "The road to hell is paved with good intentions." Good intentions can never re-purpose sin or be license for sin. We cannot abuse alcohol or steal and cheat and then protest that we intended it for God's glory. Paul asked, Shall we sin so that grace shall increase? Never. Our theme verse for engaging in Christian yoga is 1 Thessalonians 5:21-22: "Test everything. Hold on to the good. Avoid every kind of evil."

What is mysticism? Can mysticism be Christian? Isn't yoga mystical?

Yoga is not necessarily mystical except that in Christian yoga, we have our relationship with God at the center. Simply put, mysticism is seeking communication with and experience of the supernatural or divine. At the heart of the Christian faith is a mystical connection. Humanity is invited into relationship with God who has revealed himself as both supernatural and divine by his very nature. Any relationship includes communication and experience. How can the pursuit of life in Christ be anything but mystical?

Shouldn't we call it something different than Christian yoga?

Language constantly evolves. New words are added all the time and old words acquire new meanings and usages. C.S. Lewis described language as a living tree, constantly sending out new limbs and branches.[5] To "google" is now an accepted and widely used verb. Some words that we use today had original meanings that were the exact opposite of their intended meaning today. Consider the word *terrific,* which we now use to describe something that is *fabulous* or *wonderful* when it originally meant *horrifying* or *terrifying.*

In a similar way the word *yoga* in our western society has changed and now represents a narrower reference than it originally did. There is evidence of this narrowing of meaning in the widely published concern of Hindu yogis that *yoga* is merely understood as a physical practice of health in the west. It is not unreasonable to suggest that *yoga* as a word has entered the English lexicon with a new meaning acquired in a western context. This meaning is now unique from what *yoga* may have initially represented within an eastern or Hindu religious context.

A strong precedent exists for developing and establishing unique schools and styles of yoga, especially in America. Each of these schools has their own unique sets of postures and specific emphases. Some of these are Bikram yoga, Iyengar yoga, Anusara yoga, Ashtanga yoga, Yoga Fit, power yoga, hot yoga, kid yoga and pet yoga (yes it's true). These schools have some things in common but differ greatly on others. Similarly, we can call Christian yoga a new school of yoga with different and unique philosophies.

With all of this in mind, it is not insincere to call the practice Christian *yoga* while not embracing the cultural and religious context through which it came to us. Calling it *Christian* also distinguishes it from other yoga. Since Christian yoga does employ specific physical practices that anyone would recognize as yoga, it would be disingenuous to call it something else.

Who is Patanjali and what is the Eight-fold Path?

Patanjali is often described as the father of yoga. Sometime between 300 BC and 300 AD Patanjali wrote the Yoga Sutras. He was the first known person to organize and write down a philosophy of yoga even though we saw that there is evidence that yoga had already been practiced for a few thousand years. Patanjali laid out the Eight-fold Path as a prescription for living with a clear list of what to do and what not to do. The first two steps are lists of abstinences and observances:

Patanjali's Abstinences
No violence, No lying, No stealing, No lust, No greed
Patanjali's Observances
Purity, Contentment, Self-discipline, Study (of self and scriptures), Devotion to God

The eight-fold path also includes body control, breath control, detachment, concentration and meditation.[6]

Many of these precepts are very biblical exhortations. The Ten Commandments tell us not to murder, lie or steal. Greed and lust are repeatedly identified as sin and we are instructed to be pure, content and self disciplined. Study of the Bible, examination of the heart and devotion to God should characterize every believer's life. In the Old Testament God commanded Joshua, "Do not let this Book of the Law depart from your mouth; *meditate* on it day and night, so that you may be careful to do everything written in it. Then you will be prosperous and successful." Following many of Patanjali's rules and following the Bible's rules are very similar and would benefit anyone. But we have to ask ourselves if following external rules has the power to change our hearts.

There is a key difference between Patanjali and the Bible that the Christian cannot ignore. The eighth step in Patanjali's path is the achievement of bliss or *Samadhi*; in other words, salvation. Patanjali promises that by living according to this path we will save ourselves. In contrast, the Bible says that we will live this way because of God's gracious saving work in our life that starts when we choose to follow Christ, the Way, the Truth and the Life. Where is your trust? In your own ability to follow the rules? Or in the saving grace of God that transforms your heart?

Time to catch our breath! We've completed our whirlwind tour considering the questions about Christian yoga. Here is a brief recap:

1. Our worldview defines our motivation for and the nature of our Christian yoga practice. Our worldview includes our assumptions about who we are, about the world around us and how we relate to it, and what we believe about God.

2. Our heart and intentions give our practice its meaning.

3. Yoga is a method not a theology. Our theology defines how this method is used.

When our worldview, intentions and theology are grounded in the Word of God and we keep our practice centered on Christ, we honor God.

I hope you are excited about the possibilities of Christian yoga as a way to pursue the kind of self-care we've discussed. Self-care motivated by a primary regard for God and others is radical! Outwardly oriented self-care is counter cultural today. But our outward orientation has to have its origin in inward focus first. We have to spend time *being* before we get too busy *doing*. We start with tending to our soul.

[1] Nirmala Heriza, *Dr. Yoga: Yoga for Health*, (New York: Jeremy P. Tarcher/Penguin, 2004), p. xxi.

[2] Pantheism is the belief that God is everything and everything is God. Monism is the belief that there is only one whole ultimate reality without any independent parts, therefore there is no distinction to be made between you and I or anything.

[3] Psalm 118:24, Lamentations 3:22-23, Malachi 4:2

[4] Tilden Edwards in the Foreword to Nancy Roth, *An Invitation to Christian Yoga*, (New York: Seabury Books, 2005), p.xii.

[5] C.S. Lewis, *Miracles*, (Glasgow: Fount Paperbacks, 1987), p.175.

[6] Joan Budilovsky and Eve Adamson, *The Complete Idiot's Guide to Yoga*, 2nd ed, (Indianapolis: Alpha Books, 2001), p. 67.

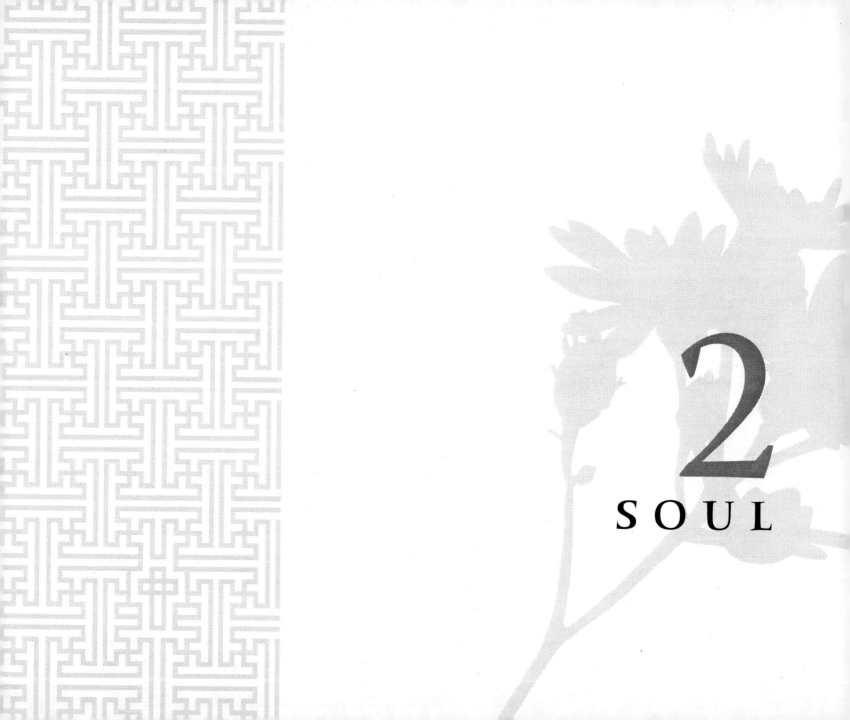

2
SOUL

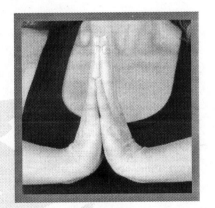 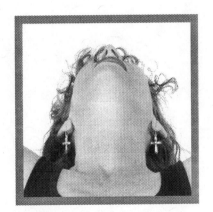 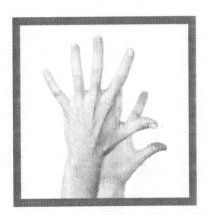

*My soul yearns
and even faints,
for the courts of the Lord;
my heart and flesh cry out for
the living God.*
PSALM 84:2

CHAPTER FOUR

Hungry & Thirsty

MY HEART WAS going to explode. I knew it. I looked down at the downy headed alien who had just invaded my world and totally surrendered. A fierce love overwhelmed me. My heart did crack open and I discovered a capacity for joy and delight that I never knew existed. Motherhood engulfed me. Nothing was left unchanged.

At times of such incredible emotion and response we wonder at the depth and origin of these feelings. Somehow we know that we have caught a glimpse of something far greater than what we know here on earth.

We feel the same mystery when overcome with sadness and grief over evil and injustice. Surely this is not what God intended. Surely we were made for something more than this, something different. Life in this fallen world doesn't fit us perfectly and we chafe uncomfortably, longing for freedom. Longing for something we can't quite name. There is an emptiness, a hollowness inside us much like hunger in our stomachs.

Augustine of Hippo, at the very beginning of his *Confessions*, declared to God, "You made us for Yourself; and our heart is restless until it finds rest in You."[1] We do have restless hearts. This inner restlessness is particularly evident in our consumer driven society today. At the heart of our conspicuous consumption lies the hope that we will actually find happiness and satisfaction that will quiet this discontent. Blaise Pascal also wrote of this inner longing:

My soul yearns for you in the night; in the morning my spirit longs for you.
ISAIAH 26:9

As the deer pants for streams of water, so my soul pants for you, O God.
My soul thirsts for God, for the living God.
When can I go and meet with God?
PSALM 42:1-2

What is it then, that this desire and this inability (to satisfy it) proclaim to us, but that there was once in man a true happiness of which there now remain to him only the mark and empty trace, which he in vain tries to fill from all his surroundings, seeking from things absent the help he does not obtain in things present? But these are all inadequate, because the infinite abyss can only be filled by an infinite and immutable object, that is to say, only by God himself. [2]

The popular idea of a "God-shaped hole" that exists in each of us originated with this thought from Pascal. The truth is we are made in God's image and there is hardwired into our souls a holy discontent with life in this fallen world. Ecclesiastes 3:11 says that God "set eternity in the hearts of men." With the memory of Eden in our hearts we long for God. Our souls hunger and thirst for God just as David cried out from the desert of Judah:

O God, you are my God, earnestly I seek you;

my soul thirsts for you, my body longs for you,

in a dry and weary land

where there is no water (Psalm 63:1).

A baby's cry signals to her mother her hunger and thirst, her most basic needs. When we care for our souls, we start with recognizing our most basic spiritual needs: the hunger and thirst for God.

Come, Eat and Drink

God knows intimately the deep hunger and thirst of our souls because he made us. He invites us to come to him and find true satisfaction. Listen to this beautiful invitation:

> Come, all you who are thirsty, come to the waters;
>
> and you who have no money, come, buy and eat!
>
> Come, buy wine and milk without money and without cost.
>
> Why spend money on what is not bread, and your labor on what does not satisfy?
>
> Listen, listen to me, and eat what is good,
>
> and your soul will delight in the richest of fare.
>
> Give ear and come to me; hear me, that your soul may live.
>
> I will make an everlasting covenant with you,
>
> my faithful love promised to David (Isaiah 55:1-3).

God alone can satisfy our soul's hunger and thirst. He promises that when we seek him, we will find him; that when we come to him to be filled instead of trying to feed our discontent with the things of this world, that we will feast on "the richest of fare"—on fabulous soul food we can't even imagine.

In order to live, we need to eat. Otherwise we starve and become emaciated. We need food but it must be quality food for our bodies to grow in strength and health. Our souls need to be fed too. Is your soul malnourished, starving or stunted? Your soul can thrive and flourish, feasting on quality food. We feed our souls like this by listening to God. He says, "hear me, *that your soul may live.*" Jesus gave a similar invitation in John 6:35, "I am the bread of life. He who comes to me will never go hungry, and he who believes in me will never be thirsty." This is where we find true satisfaction of our inner restlessness.

When we fill ourselves with God we cannot stay unchanged. Later in Isaiah chapter 55 God tells us that his ways and his thoughts are not the same as our thoughts and ways; his are so much higher than ours. This does not mean that they are inaccessible to us. Instead, he calls us to forsake our thoughts and ways and *replace* them with his. The more we spend time with God the more we begin to think like him and to act like him. This on-going exchange is at the heart of our transformation or our spirituality.[3]

An Authentic Christian Spirituality

These days, religion is out but spirituality is in.
KENNETH BOA
CONFORMED TO HIS IMAGE

The hunger for something bigger than ourselves is so evident in the current spiritual temperature. Spirituality is a very popular word these days. Many people prefer to identify themselves as spiritual rather than as religious. "Religious" seems to infer rigidity, intolerance and dogma, while "spiritual" may acknowledge a belief in something beyond our tangible experience but perhaps an unwillingness to define it or declare any objective truth about it. Society's openness to this generic kind of spirituality explains much of the broad appeal and current popularity of yoga and eastern religious traditions.

My introduction to Christian yoga intersected a personal journey of exploration of questions about spiritual formation. For a number of years I had been reading about and wrestling with the questions of how to "work out my salvation", how to "offer my body as a living sacrifice" and how it is that I am transformed into the likeness of Christ and can grow in grace. Spiritual formation is the name put to the process through which these things happen, the process through which Christ is formed in us and we are conformed to his image. God does this transforming work in our lives once we have placed our trust in Christ but he calls us to cooperate with him in the process. In my exploration of writing and teachings on spiritual formation I was introduced to the spiritual disciplines. These disciplines are things that we do as part of our cooperation with God in our formation in Christ.

Discipline is not necessarily an attractive word to many of us. I have struggled my whole life to develop greater self-discipline in so many areas and probably will keep struggling. But it is worth striving for because discipline is an essential part of the Christian life. "Discipline yourselves for the purpose of godliness," Timothy tells us.[4] One definition I was given for spiritual discipline is "any activity that helps me gain power to live life as Jesus taught and modeled it." I like that. I can work with that.

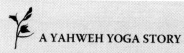

A YAHWEH YOGA STORY

Practicing Christ centered yoga has changed my life. I am a Christian psychologist, author and speaker and am well informed on the benefits of self care.

For years I worked out at a local gym and tolerated the music that was toxic to my soul. Two years ago following a routine of weights and squats I tore the meniscus in my knee. During recovery from surgery I asked the Lord to reveal a healthful way to exercise, appropriate for my age and conducive to my soul.

Following this prayer request I was asked to speak at a Spa for the Soul retreat in the Midwest. That weekend I was introduced to Christ-centered yoga. I was awed and amazed at the integrative approach to physical and spiritual health. But could I find something like that at home?

The spiritual disciplines are many and the lists vary with the authors who write about them. Some of the disciplines are prayer, worship, confession, solitude, meditation, stewardship, silence and simplicity. Pursuing the disciplines is about the inward condition of our hearts, not about mastering an outward display of spirituality. We can only undertake these disciplines in the context of God's grace. Richard Foster describes the disciplines as "penetrated throughout by the enabling grace of God."[5]

When I was introduced to Christian yoga I saw a beautiful potential for the integration of the disciplines of yoga with the pursuit of the grace-enabled, spiritually disciplined life. When yoga is applied in a Christian context with all the considerations we have already discussed it can be considered a spiritual discipline that contributes to our spiritual formation. Our spiritual formation in Christ requires that we pay close attention to the condition of our souls.

Tending to our souls is an integral part of the authentic Christian spiritual life. Regular attention to our soul helps brings us in alignment with God's will and purpose. Indeed, one of the things that is most attractive about yoga for the Christian is the priority it places on looking after your soul and the space and time it creates to pursue the inner aspects of our spirituality in Christ.

What is our soul?

I find Dallas Willard's discussion and definition of human nature in *Renovation of the Heart* the most helpful in considering what our soul is. Willard describes six aspects of human life: thought, feeling, choice, body, social context and soul. The soul is the part that integrates and inter-relates all these aspects into the whole person — it is the organizing factor.[6] Willard goes on to relate our *person* to our *pursuit* of the spiritual life and spiritual formation:

> The ideal of the spiritual life in the Christian understanding is one where all of the essential parts of the human self are effectively organized around God, as they are restored and sustained by him. *Spiritual formation in Christ is the* process *leading to that ideal end, and its result is the love of God with all of the heart, soul, mind and strength and of the neighbor as oneself.* The human self is then fully integrated under God."[7]

Here Willard has expressed our self-care goal: we want to be lovers of God and people. We see a synergy between the emphasis in hatha yoga on integrated health of the whole person and the pursuit of an integrated life under God through spiritual formation. When we take the **practice** of hatha yoga with its emphasis on physical health, self-examination and meditation and marry it with the **theory** of spiritual formation and sound

I continued to pray, search the web, interact with other ministries and a friend told me about Yahweh Yoga. It was a 20 minute drive from my home but I was compelled to go. During my first visit I knew I was experiencing an answer to my prayer. The lyrics of the music, focus on scripture, calming prayer time and caring atmosphere were more than I could ever imagine for an ongoing exercise program. I made a new set of friends who loved the Lord and valued physical, spiritual and emotional health.

My Christ-centered yoga practice has become a sacred rhythm in my week. It is a time-out to slow down, gain perspective, worship the Lord and reap the health benefits of age appropriate exercise. Recently the studio moved two miles from my home. Can you imagine my smile?
—Carol

doctrine about who we are and who God is, we have Christian yoga — an ideal means for self-care, an ideal support to the pursuit of Christian spirituality and intimacy with our Creator. The most important part of our self-care is tending to our soul. We care for our soul because it is what keeps us "fully integrated under God."

Caring for our Soul

We take our first step in soul care when we willingly respond to the invitation God extends to us to *come*. Christ's now familiar invitation to rest in Matthew chapter 11 echoes the invitation of Isaiah 55. Here it is again but this time in the words of *The Message:*

> Are you tired? Worn out? Burned out on religion? Come to me. Get away with me and you'll recover your life. I'll show you how to take a real rest. Walk with me and work with me—watch how I do it. Learn the unforced rhythms of grace. I won't lay anything heavy or ill-fitting on you. Keep company with me and you'll learn to live freely and lightly.

Get away with me... learn the unforced rhythms of grace. How inviting. How refreshing. I want to sign up for that retreat.

We start with surrendering our baggage and burdens. This includes our expectations about what God would require of us. So many of us are reluctant to come to God without having "it all together" first. God's invitation is to come buy and eat *without money*. In other words, come as you are. Come only with your hunger and thirst and your weariness. A broken and contrite heart is the only offering God desires. You don't need to pay for your place at the table; come empty-handed and trusting, like the children that Jesus said His kingdom belonged to.

We come to the Lord by placing ourselves in his presence, by *getting away* with him. Although we know that God can meet us anywhere, when we create a sanctuary in our hearts we can hear him speak to us so much better. We can respond to God's invitation to come into his presence through being intentional about our environment. We do that by seeking silence and solitude.

[1] Saint Augustine, *Confessions* 1.1 (author's paraphrase of translation by Edward Bouverie Pusey.)

[2] Blaise Pascal, *Pensées* Section 7, 425.

[3] I am grateful to Pastor Sunder Krishnan, for his beautiful and thoughtful exposition of Isaiah 55 in his message series, "Living as Called People in Driven World."

[4] 1 Timothy 4:7

[5] Richard Foster, "Spiritual Formation: A Pastoral Letter," *The Ooze*, *http://www.theooze.com/articles/article.cfm?id=744* (July 24, 2006).

[6] Dallas Willard, *Renovation of the Heart*, (Colorado Springs: NavPress, 2002), p.30.

[7] Willard, p. 31.

CHAPTER FIVE

Be Still

SILENCE AND SOLITUDE. Doesn't that sound inviting? Or maybe it sounds scary to you. Finding solitude or even desiring to seek it can be extraordinarily difficult. We are bombarded with noise and busyness all the time and many of us are conditioned to it. It's our normal mode. Real silence can be deafening and real solitude threatening. Not everyone is comfortable just hanging out with herself. We need to unlearn habits of noise and endless activity, both in our environment and in our heads, and listen to Christ's invitation to "Come away with me to a quiet place…"

Noise comes to us in many ways, some not always recognized. A number of years ago we moved with our family to Thailand to live in Bangkok, a messy, polluted, overwhelming metropolis buzzing with human activity. We had left a quiet suburban life in Canada in exchange for an urban life filled with sensory overload. Even in our high rise condo we could not completely escape the noise and pollution. Something was always humming and running. There was a certain thrill to the constant activity and hustle and bustle of humanity but it wore us down.

We learned from seasoned expatriates the importance of regularly escaping the city to the quieter beach towns and resorts in order to remove ourselves from the constant demand and stress on our systems. However, we came to appreciate a different aspect of quiet that came with living in a foreign culture. Because we could speak very little Thai our ability to understand the incessant input around us was limited. Any junk mail we

The Lord is in his holy temple;
let all the earth be silent before him.
HABAKKUK 2:20

There is a time for everything,
a season for every activity
* under heaven…a time to be silent*
and a time to speak…
ECCLESIASTES 3:17

Be still and know that I am God.
PSALM 46:10

received was in Thai. We chose not to have cable TV and were limited to one Australian station in English. The Wiggles and Aussie cooking shows were our only television options. Radio was in Thai, billboards were in Thai. Being cut off by language created a different kind of reduction in noise, a different kind of space in our heads. My husband called it "mindspace".

When we moved back to North America, I was overwhelmed by the constant barrage of communication demanding my attention. My mailbox now overflows with flyers, special offers and magazines. Television choices are endless. Radio stations to suit every taste and political leaning are abundant. I am constantly confronted with language I can understand—I can read the billboards, the bus shelters, the signs, all the product labels. Both wittingly and unwittingly I am subject to constant mental input. While my external environment may be quieter and less demanding, my internal environment is far more taxed. The paradox of Bangkok was that I had a different kind of space for time with God in the midst of crazy and exhausting circumstances.

Silence and solitude are among the traditional disciplines of our faith. In exercising the disciplines of silence and solitude there are two aspects to consider. First, we need to place ourselves in a silent environment, cutting off external noise and distraction. Then, we need to choose to be silent ourselves, quieting the inner noise and being still before God.

Our desire for and comfort in silence and solitude will be influenced by our temperament. If you are an introvert, being alone energizes you and you probably already naturally seek out solitude. I am not like that. I am more of an extrovert and I can find solitude and silence very challenging. Although, the older I get, the more I crave it and need it. But I have to make conscious choices and plan carefully to make it happen. With any spiritual discipline, you will be drawn more to some than others because of your temperament. It is important not to just stay where we are comfortable but to challenge and stretch ourselves in new ways. Dietrich Bonhoeffer wrote of the twin importance of solitude and fellowship and warned:

> Let him who cannot be alone beware of community...Let him who is not in community beware of being alone....One who wants fellowship without solitude plunges into the void of words and feelings and one who seeks solitude without fellowship perishes in the abyss of vanity, self-infatuation and despair.[1]

There are numerous biblical reasons for pursuing quiet time alone. In silence we hear the voice of God better, express faith and trust in him, and are physically and emotionally restored. I believe the most compelling reason is to follow Jesus' example. Repeatedly in the gospels we see Jesus retreating from the crowds, rising before dawn, sending the disciples on ahead, all in order to meet with his Father and pray. The demands of his ministry made solitude a necessity.

One of my favorite examples is in chapter six of the gospel of Mark. Jesus' disciples returned from being sent out to preach by him, all flushed with exhilaration over the things they have done and seen. They had driven out demons, miraculously healed people and preached repentance! I can just imagine them trying to talk all at once in their excitement. They had taken no provisions with them and were probably running on adrenaline. The scene is described this way: "there were so many people coming and going that they did not even have a chance to eat" (v. 31). I don't know about you but that description is painfully familiar. The disciples just had their first taste of independent and powerful ministry and now they were feeling the toll on their bodies. Jesus invited them to follow his example, "Come with me by yourselves to a quiet place and get some rest." *This is what you need to do if you are going to continue to minister in power and in my name.*

Quiet time alone with God helps us both recover from and prepare for ministry. As with self-care in general, solitude is not an end in itself. We seek it in order to be better able to serve. Jesus and his disciples were not alone for very long. They withdrew to a boat but the crowd followed them on shore, clamoring for their attention. That is also very familiar. As a mom, finding any space alone is a challenge. Even if I am in the bathroom, there will often be little fingers reaching under the door and a little voice calling, "Mommy, are you in there? Can I come in too? When are you coming out?" It says that when they landed on the shore, Jesus had compassion on the crowds and began to teach them, because they were "like sheep without a shepherd." And Jesus went on to feed this crowd of thousands with a meager five bread rolls and two fish! The moment you step out of your quiet place, everyone will be clamoring for you but you will be far better equipped to rise to the challenges before you with compassion and grace.

What are some practical ways to integrate solitude into our lives?

If this is a challenge for you, find small ways to begin. Maybe you have some habits of noise that you can begin to undo. Try not turning on the television just because you are in the room. Drive in the car without the radio on. Take a walk without your iPod. During a solitary meal resist the temptation to read a magazine or book. Take baby steps.

From there, you can move to being more intentional about finding solitude. Set the alarm early to wake up before the rest of the house. Create a space in your home, whether it is just a chair or an entire room, where you can be alone. (I have read somewhere that Susannah Wesley, mother of ten living children, would sit down in a chair by the fire and pull an apron over her head, a sign to all to leave mama alone to pray.) You could also consider planning a silent retreat. Try withdrawing from your world for a day or a weekend to be quiet before God.

With solitude and silence being a challenge to achieve in our busy lives, take advantage of the regular practice of Christian yoga to create sanctuary for your soul. I know many

truly a place where for an hour you can completely relinquish the cares of the world. The practice encourages me to calm down my mind from constant overdrive, and focus on the Lord. I find I leave the class with a more positive attitude, sense of deep gratitude and a spring in my step. After evening classes I sleep really well.

I truly feel Yahweh Yoga is a holy place. We all gather together from different churches to praise and worship the living God. The nature of the practice allows us to find solitude and just be with Our Lord. The scripture readings before and after are so meaningful and set the stage for the practice. The lovely Christian music is a further aid to develop a sense of peace and oneness with the Lord.

So often it seems as though the scriptures read are chosen just for me and minister to some need I currently have in my life. I have come to treasure the time I can spend in these classes.

- Claudia

Christians who have designated their yoga mat a sacred space. It is helpful to have a tangible expression and boundary of solitude like this. Even in a class setting, yoga is a solo practice. Don't pay attention to others around you and close your eyes as much as possible. Sink into your own solitude to prepare yourself for a time of meditation and self-examination, to feed your soul.

We have created a sanctuary for our soul and we have entered into God's presence. Now we need to listen for his voice and examine our hearts.

[1] As quoted in Richard J. Foster, *Celebration of Discipline: The Path to Spiritual Growth*, 20th Anniversary ed., (San Francisco: HarperSanFrancisco, 1998), p.97.

CHAPTER SIX

Meditation

ONE OF CHRISTIAN yoga's greatest benefits is how it creates an environment for meditation and sets an imperative for deliberate focus and intention of the mind. To meditate means to think deeply or to focus one's mind for a period of time. It also means to think carefully about something. Many Christians are uncomfortable with meditation. Some believe it to be a dangerous opening of the mind to unknown forces. Indeed, in New Age practices, meditation is linked with connecting with spirit guides. Christians are also rightly concerned about the eastern intentions of emptying your mind and detaching from self and from the world. But meditation is very much a Christian and biblical practice too. Christian meditation is unique from these other forms, however, in very important ways that we will examine here.

We already looked briefly at disciplined spirituality—meditation is one of the key spiritual disciplines. There are many books on Christian spiritual formation and I think it is safe to say that meditation is included in them all. Richard Foster writes one of the clearest explanations of the differences between eastern meditation and Christian meditation:

> Eastern meditation is an attempt to empty the mind. Christian meditation is an attempt to fill the mind. The two ideas are quite different. Eastern forms of meditation stress the need to become detached from the world. There is an emphasis on losing personhood and individuality and merging with the Cosmic Mind. There is a longing to be freed from the burden and pains of this life and to

Oh, how I love your law! I meditate on it all day long.
PSALM 119:97

May the words of my mouth and the meditation of my heart be pleasing in your sight, O LORD, my Rock and my Redeemer.
PSALM 19:14

be released into the impersonality of Nirvana. Personal identity is lost and, in fact, personality is seen as the ultimate illusion. There is no escaping from the miserable wheel of existence. There is no God to be attached to or to hear from. Detachment is the final goal of Eastern religion.

Christian meditation goes far beyond the notion of detachment...No, detachment is not enough; we must go on to attachment. The detachment from the confusion all around us is in order to have a richer attachment to God. Christian meditation leads us to the inner wholeness necessary to give ourselves to God freely.[1]

Foster acknowledges the need for detachment but it is an entirely different concept with a different purpose than the eastern notion. My youngest son always seems to be clamoring for my attention when I can give it to him the least—in that brief window of chaos between school and dinner. I will be on the phone, making supper, changing laundry and managing homework with my older two and he is yanking on my arm and talking louder and louder, in the hopes that I will hear him. There are too many competing demands for my attention and at that time of day he loses out. But because he is the youngest by a number of years we have a lot of time at home alone together. Since he was tiny we have had a precious time after lunch of stories and cuddles—just mommy and him, no distractions, nothing else that is more important. That is my picture of detachment—a deliberate setting apart and removal from distractions and competing demands for my attention so that I can focus on God.

Empty or Full?

The contrast between emptying and filling is also an important distinction between eastern and Christian meditation. We may make an attempt to empty our minds of distracting thoughts, however, it is always for the purpose of being filled with the thoughts of God. *Empty* is rarely used in a positive sense. It indicates a lack, a vacuum, a void, or an absence. In the Bible we find *empty-handed, empty-headed, an empty land, empty words, empty thoughts, empty pursuits, empty hearts, empty souls, empty lives.* In *The Message*, Eugene Peterson replaces the word *fool* with *empty-head.*

I really don't want to be an empty-head. Instead I want to "be filled to the measure of all the fullness of God."[2] I want to be given a good measure of God, pressed down, shaken together and running over. We used to sing a Sunday school song that went "running over, running over, my cup is full and running over" from Psalm 23. Emptiness does not draw me. No, I want my heart to overflow with joy, thankfulness, hope, love, and praise because it has been filled with God so full that bitterness, malice, rage, anger, hate, despair and sin have been flooded out. I believe that Jesus came so that I "might have life and have it to the *full*" (John 10:10).

As followers of Christ we are called to a life of transformation not vacancy. We are transformed by the renewing of our mind, which is accomplished by God's Word and His Spirit.

> Since you have heard about Jesus and have learned the truth that comes from him, throw off your old sinful nature and your former way of life, which is corrupted by lust and deception. Instead, let the Spirit renew your thoughts and attitudes. Put on your new nature, created to be like God—truly righteous and holy (Ephesians 4:21-24).

If our meditation is to be a transforming discipline that renews our minds it must be grounded in the Bible. Kenneth Boa stresses the extreme importance of God's Word as the anchor of our meditation to guard against phony or occult practices:

> Meditation and contemplation must always be tethered to the truth of the Word. Contemplation is not an introspective New Age practice of altered consciousness or voiding the mind of content. Engagement in bogus mysticism and introspection leads at best to sloppy sentimentality and self delusion and at worst to demonic influences. We circumvent this dangerous territory *by commitment to sound doctrine, by being comfortable with a high view of Scripture, and by approaching the Word with a willingness to study it and put it in practice.* [3]

So when we approach meditation as Christians, we anchor ourselves in Scripture, we seek to remove ourselves from distraction in order to fully attend to God and we ask him to fill us. Our purpose in meditation is to grow deeper into our relationship and understanding of God. We want to think deeply, think carefully and focus on Him.

Listening

When we considered how we tend to our soul, we saw that we need to come and we need to listen. Meditation is an important means of helping us to listen for God's voice. He speaks to us in many ways but unless we are listening we will miss his calling and his leading. One of my favorite stories is found in chapter nineteen of 1 Kings.

Elijah has just hosted a spectacular showdown between God and the prophets of Baal. God showed himself mighty and the idols and their prophets were destroyed. Although Elijah was triumphant, he is now on the run from Jezebel, who has vowed to destroy him. After days on foot through the desert, Elijah finds himself in a cave in the middle of nowhere. God comes to him and asks him, "What are you doing here, Elijah?" You can hear the weariness, fatigue and perhaps even hopelessness in Elijah's reply: *I'm the only one who is really serving you God. Everyone else has rejected you and killed your prophets and they want to kill me too. What do you think I am doing? I am running away!*

God speaks to him again and tells him to leave the cave and stand in the presence of the LORD, for the LORD is about to pass by. Then a powerful wind shakes the mountains apart, but God is not in the wind. After the wind, there is an earthquake, but God is not in the earthquake. Then a great fire burns, but God is not in the fire. And then after the fire, there comes a gentle whisper. It is when he hears this whisper, that Elijah covers his head and finally steps out of the cave, into the presence of the LORD.

Don't we sometimes wish God would speak to us in thunderous, spectacular ways? I would like God to speak very loudly and clearly to me. I wouldn't even mind if everyone else heard him do it. Most of the time, however, God chooses to speak to us in a whisper, in a still small voice, in the promptings of our heart, through his Word. Unless we are listening carefully, we will miss it. We start meditation in the sanctuary we have created through silence and solitude. *Be still and know that I am God.* Then we heed the advice of Solomon in Ecclesiastes and we listen.

> Guard your steps when you go to the house of God. Go near to listen rather than to offer the sacrifice of fools, who do not know that they do wrong. Do not be quick with your mouth, do not be hasty in your heart to utter anything before God. God is in heaven and you are on earth, so let your words be few (Ecclesiastes 5:1-2).

What do we meditate on?

After Moses died Joshua took over the command of Israel. At the beginni

command, God gave him some very specific promises and instructions which

these words: "Do not let this Book of the Law depart from your mouth; meditate o

and night, so that you may be careful to do everything written in it. Then you w

prosperous and successful" (Joshua 1:8). Joshua's success as leader of Israel depende

his commitment to God's Word and his obedience to it. Meditation is one of the ways

take our head knowledge and move it into heart wisdom so we can work it out i

obedience.

In the Bible, we find this specific command to meditate, many other passages that

commend the same practice but with a different name *(consider, think on, remember, listen)*

and numerous examples of meditation modeled for us, particularly in the Psalms. There

are three primary subjects for our meditation.

We Meditate on God

God's "unfailing love" is one of his attributes or qualities, as is the "glorious splendor of his

majesty." We start with meditating on God and who he is. In the opening chapter of

Knowledge of the Holy, A.W. Tozer states, " What comes into our minds when we think

about God is the most important thing about us...Worship is pure or base as the

May my meditation be pleasing to him, as I rejoice in the LORD.
PSALM 104:34

They will speak of the glorious splendor of your majesty, and I will meditate on your wonderful works.
PSALM 145:5

Within your temple, O God, we meditate on your unfailing love.
PSALM 48:9

worshipper entertains high or low thoughts of God...We tend by a secret law of the soul to move toward our mental image of God."[4] God has revealed so much about himself through Scripture. We know his different names, all communicating some truth about his nature, and we know what he says about himself.

If you have never studied the names or attributes of God, this is an excellent place to begin your meditation. Just through his names, we know that God is the Creator, the Most High, the God who sees, the All-Sufficient One, the Master, our Healer, our Provider, Peace, our Shepherd, our Righteousness—there are more. Don't these names invite you to spend time considering what their significance is for you? When we contemplate who God is and meditate on his nature, we will be confronted with his "otherness", his holiness, and say with the Psalmist, "Who is like the Lord?" Not me.

We Meditate on His Word

Psalm 119 records a love affair of the Psalmist with God's Word. The Psalmist speaks of God's law and his promises. He rejoices in them, delights in them, learns them, hides them in his heart, seeks them, desires them, speaks of them, obeys them and considers and meditates on them. Eleven times he cries out to God "preserve my life!" according to your word, your love, your statutes, your promises. God's Word is our life, it is our daily bread. When Moses finished declaring God's law to Israel in the book of Deuteronomy, he

I meditate on your precepts and consider your ways.
PSALM 119:15

I lift up my hands to your commands, which I love, and I meditate on your decrees.
PSALM 119:48

My eyes stay open through the watches of the night, that I may meditate on your promises.
PSALM 119:148

But his delight is in the law of the LORD, and on his law he meditates day and night.
PSALM 1:2

warned them to take it very seriously: "These are not just idle words for you—*these are your life.*"[5] We need to ingest God's Word daily, and then digest it, meditate and ruminate upon it, and receive the power and energy to live that it offers. Psalm 119:11 says, "I have hidden your word in my heart that I might not sin against you." We are hiding God's laws in our heart to direct us and his promises to give us hope.

We should be familiar with the passages that we meditate on. It is helpful and important to understand context and meaning prior to meditating. This is why Bible study is an important discipline that should also be pursued with meditation. Meditation is not Bible study but it is greatly aided by it. You don't need a complete and deeply exegetical understanding of Scripture prior to meditating on it but you do need to have a reasonable grasp of it. A high view of Scripture means that we guard against manipulating it to suit our purposes. "Let me understand the teaching of your precepts; *then* I will meditate on your wonders" (Psalm 119:27).

When you meditate on Scripture, start with a short portion, a verse or two. Begin with prayer, asking God to move His word from your head into your heart. Read it aloud or listen to it being read. Then ponder it slowly and carefully in your heart, resisting the temptation to rush through. Examine the words, imagine the circumstances, consider how you feel in response to it, ask God to show you what your response should be. Turn the Scripture into a personalized prayer back to God. You may be convicted of sin or inaction, you may be overwhelmed with praise and worship, or you may need to pray for grace and courage to act upon what God is teaching you.

Two formal approaches to Scripture meditation that have been developed and used by Christians are *lectio divina* (sacred reading) and formational Scripture reading. In formational reading you primarily change your perspective of God's Word from being a text to master to instead being a text that masters you and works on your spirit and soul, forming Christ within you. When we come to Scripture with this attitude we are believing that God's Word is "living and active" in us and transforming us.

The formational method is very similar to lectio divina which is an approach to Scripture that originated with the desert fathers and mothers in the 4th century. It has four steps or elements, described in Latin as *lectio* (reading), *meditatio* (meditation), *oratio* (prayer) and *contemplatio* (contemplation). The four steps are fairly self-explanatory. You start with slowly and carefully reading a portion of Scripture. You then spend some time reflecting on the passage. After internalizing the Scripture you return it to the Lord in prayer. The final stage is resting and silence in the presence of God, in communion with him.

A student once shared a vernacular version of lectio divina which I have appreciated. I can just imagine an old time country preacher pounding his fist in the pulpit and proclaiming this:

I reads myself full.

I thinks myself clear.

I prays myself hot!

I lets myself go.

These different methods and approaches to meditating on Scripture can be very helpful but be careful not to merely practice a method. Feel free to adapt these elements for yourself. Don't be rigid in your application but instead move freely back and forth between these steps. This is a personal process and time with God. When we hide his Word in our hearts, it will keep us from sin; when we feed our soul on the bread of life, we will hunger no more.

We Meditate on His Works

In the Psalms we see examples of meditation on God himself, meditation on his word, and also meditation on his works, what he has done and what he is doing still. This could be called a meditation of remembering. In Psalm 77, Asaph is crying out in distress. He is groaning and in the anguished state of believing that God has forsaken him. "Will the Lord reject forever? Has his unfailing love vanished forever?" In the midst of his pain, he makes a choice and declares, "To this I will appeal: the years of the right hand of the Most

I will meditate on all your works and consider all your mighty deeds.
PSALM 77:12

I remember the days of long ago; I meditate on all your works and consider what your hands have done.
PSALM 143:5

High. I will remember the deeds of the Lord: yes I will remember your miracles of long ago. *I will meditate on all your works and consider all your mighty deeds"* (v.10-12). At this point, the Psalm changes from pain and anguish to singing praise and recounting God's mighty works and faithfulness to Israel. When we choose to remember what God has done, whether it is from the Bible, or what he has done in our own life or others, it takes our focus off our circumstances and fills us with hope and confidence in His ability and faithfulness to continue to do mighty deeds in our life. The change in focus is simple but has profound implications for us.

The most visible evidence of God's mighty works is in his creation. We can meditate on beauty and power in nature. Living in the desert, I have seen sunsets so lovely that my heart aches watching them. I have also stood transfixed by ferocious dust and wind storms speed across the flat expanse with stunning intensity. Our family has had the privilege of seeing first-hand spectacular displays of God's creative power and genius like the Grand Canyon, the majestic Canadian Rockies, stunning coral reefs and endless beaches of the Pacific. When I am confronted with the splendor of God in creation, my heart wells up inside me and the words of the old hymn spring unbidden to my lips:

> O Lord my God, When I in awesome wonder,
> Consider all the worlds Thy Hands have made;
> I see the stars, I hear the rolling thunder,

Thy power throughout the universe displayed.

Then sings my soul, My Savior God, to Thee,

How great Thou art, How great Thou art.

Then sings my soul, My Savior God, to Thee,

How great Thou art, How great Thou art!

—CARL G. BOBERG, STUART HINE, *HOW GREAT THOU ART*

Considering creation and meditating on God's masterpieces brings us back to meditating on God himself. Romans 1:19 says, "For since the creation of the world God's invisible qualities—his eternal power and divine nature—have been clearly seen, being understood from what has been made." Meditation on creation reveals to us truth about who God is and his qualities and reminds us of who we are. We will be moved to praise just as David in Psalm 8:

When I consider your heavens,

the work of your fingers,

the moon and the stars,

which you have set in place,

what is man that you are mindful of him,

the son of man that you care for him?

...O Lord, our Lord,

how majestic is your name in all the earth!

These three are the primary subjects of our meditation: God himself, his word and his works. Other meaningful subjects of Christian meditation are devotional writings or secondary Christian writing and sacred art. So many have gone before us on this journey, whom God has used mightily and gifted with insight and the ability to convey it. Spending time with the works of these artists, writers, preachers and saints will only enrich us. They speak to us from a common earthly perspective and bring us novel insight and perspective on truth.

The Gift of Imagination

The natural ability that will enrich and enable our meditation the most is our imagination. For some reason the imagination has assumed a questionable place in some Christians' minds. Is it okay to use our imaginations when engaging with Scripture and thinking about God? I take us back to our earlier discussion about the nature of humanity. We saw that we are made by God in his image and that he declared his creation good. That means that he chose to gift us with imagination and that it is good. Surely, if he decided to give us the power of imagination, he intended that we use it. As with all the methods and approaches to meditation we must be careful to keep our imaginations anchored in truth; then they can soar in freedom without fear of being lost in the wild blue yonder, much like a kite firmly in the grasp of a child on the beach.

Not all of us are very comfortable with our imaginations but I encourage you to try using it. For example, take a story or a parable of Jesus. Imagine what it would have felt like to be a part of the crowd listening at his feet. What are the sounds you hear? What are the smells? How do his words make you feel? Or place yourself in the story as one of the main characters. Imagine that you are the woman caught in adultery and about to be stoned. Or that you are Zacchaeus, eager and anxious to see Jesus but also embarrassed, straining from your awkward perch in a tree. I promise that when you start to use your imagination you will experience a whole new dimension of God's Word and truth. Richard Foster encourages us that a sanctified imagination can be used by God to reveal truth in ways we can better comprehend it.

> To believe that God can sanctify and utilize the imagination is simply to take seriously the Christian idea of incarnation. God so accommodates, so enfleshes himself into our world that he uses the images we know and understand to teach us about the unseen world of which we know so little and which we find so difficult to understand.[6]

As a writer I am a lover of metaphor and literary devices that appeal to the imagination to communicate on a deeper, more visceral level. And I love how God invites us to use our imagination by filling His Word to us with poetry, story, drama, metaphor and symbol. It is a beautiful condescension of the unconfined Infinite to the finite frailty of our human capacities. He gifts us with our imagination and then he appeals to it—use it with joy!

Meditation and Contemplation

Meditation and contemplation are often used interchangeably as synonyms for the same practice. Other writers and thinkers define them as two different practices, closely related but distinct. Contemplation is related to engaging with Scripture but is primarily concerned with "practicing the presence of God." In the method of lectio divina meditation and contemplation are identified as different steps. It may be helpful to think of meditation as active, seeking and engaging. In contrast contemplation is passive, receiving and listening. It is not necessary to worry too much about whether you are *meditating* or *contemplating*—instead, be mindful in your time of meditation that you are both seeking and receiving, engaging and listening.

Meditation in Yoga Practice

We've looked in depth at Christian meditation as a spiritual discipline or practice. We started out by recognizing that meditation is an important part of yoga in general and a beneficial practice of Christian yoga specifically. All of these methods and principles can easily be adapted and applied to your yoga practice. If you are practicing privately, you can start with a time of Bible reading and then continue to meditate on that Scripture through your practice. You may wish to end with an extended time of quiet meditation. The method of lectio divina is especially adaptable to the progression of yoga practice.

In a class setting, time is more limited. We strongly encourage you to only practice yoga in a Christ-centered environment. Ideally, a Christian yoga class will start with a brief passage of Scripture and meditation on it from the instructor. The remainder of the class will then be oriented around this opening theme, with accompanying Christian music and continued guidance from the instructor. At the end of class, time will be provided for rest and quiet meditation. This time is often limited by following classes or constraints of the facility but you can choose to continue in meditation after the class on returning home or by choosing to go somewhere else for some continued solitude. The discipline of meditation will elevate our practice of yoga from merely care for our bodies to care for our souls—feeding them deeply on the things of God.

In Joshua 1:8 God instructs Joshua to meditate on his Law day and night, "so that you may be careful to do everything that is in it." This is the one place in the Bible that God gives a specific imperative to meditate. He also clearly states what our purpose in doing this is: to be obedient in action. We meditate on God's Word, his works, and who he is in order to move our head knowledge into heart wisdom which will then be worked out in obedience. When we spend time *being* in God's presence it will be evident in how we live our lives, in our *doing*. God also gave Joshua a promise: If you do this, "then you will be prosperous and successful." This doesn't mean that we will build a fortune and get promoted. This means that we will be successful in following and living the life he has called us to and that we will triumph over obstacles to our obedience.

We come into his presence and we listen. Through our meditation we feed our souls "on the richest of fare" and we start exchanging our thoughts for his thoughts and our ways for his ways. This process of exchange also requires that we lay our thoughts and ways out for his examination. So we move from meditation to the discipline of self-examination.

---

[1] Richard Foster, *Celebration of Discipline*, p. 20-21.
[2] Ephesians 3:19
[3] Kenneth Boa, *Conformed to His Image*, (Grand Rapids: Zondervan, 2001), p.166, emphasis added.
[4] A.W. Tozer, *Knowledge of the Holy*, (San Francisco: Harper & Row, 1961), p.1.
[5] Deuteronomy 32:47
[6] Foster, *Celebration of Discipline*, p. 26.

CHAPTER SEVEN

Search Me, Lead Me

OCTOBER IS ONE of my favorite times of year. Not because of the harvest festivals, brilliant orange pumpkins and the promise of Thanksgiving turkey coming soon. No, I love October because I can finally open my windows. The punishing heat of the Arizona summer has lifted and fresh, desert breezes blow through the rooms of my home. October is like springtime for desert dwellers. We emerge from our dark caves where we have hidden from the sun all summer long and greet our neighbors whom we haven't seen in six months. We get excited about cleaning closets and sweeping out the nooks and crannies of our homes in anticipation of the holiday season around the corner.

Similarly, we need to do a little housekeeping and sweep the cobwebs out of the corners of our soul. We can throw open the windows and let the Light shine in, bringing in fresh air and fresh perspectives. The yoga principles of self-awareness and self-examination echo the biblical commands to examine our ways, to test ourselves, to search our hearts and to confess our sin and be forgiven. In Christian yoga we not only examine ourselves but we also lay ourselves open before the Lord for his examination of our hearts. Our prayer is that of David in Psalm 139:23-24:

> Search me, O God, and know my heart; test me and know my anxious thoughts.
> See if there is any offensive way in me, and lead me in the way everlasting.

Let us examine our ways and test them and let us return to the Lord.
LAMENTATIONS 3:40

I have considered my ways and have turned my steps to your statutes.
PSALM 119:59

Test me, O Lord, and try me, examine my heart and my mind.
PSALM 26:2

Through our meditation on the Bible, we have already opened our hearts and minds for examination by it. When we fill our mind with God's Word it works to probe and search our thoughts. "For the word of God is living and active. Sharper than any double-edged sword, it penetrates even to dividing soul and spirit, joints and marrow; it judges the thoughts and attitudes of the heart" (Hebrews 4:12).

After we have filled ourselves with God's Word, we need to allow time for this soul-searching. Self-examination is not something that we can hurry through. It takes time to carefully consider our ways. It helps to be still and listen. We listen for God to speak to us in the inner promptings of our heart and conscience. Then we check these promptings against God's word to discern his voice over our own. "Let us not love with words or tongue but with actions and in truth. This then is how we know that we belong to the truth, and how we set our hearts at rest in his presence whenever our hearts condemn us. For God is greater than our hearts, and he knows everything"(1 John 3:18-20).

Sometimes we are caught in debilitating cycles of guilt and self-recrimination or self-doubt. Have I really loved God? Am I really sorry for my sin? Am I really forgiven? Objective examination of our actions against truth allows us to determine if these feelings or doubts are false or genuine. If they are false, even though we feel them deeply, we find confidence in the fact that God knows us more intimately than ourselves, that He knows *everything*, yet He freely forgives us anyway. This is why self-examination must be conducted in the context of Scripture and of listening to God, and asking him to search our hearts. If we do it merely on our own, we are in danger of getting lost in our own navels and mired in the muck of self-loathing, or being deluded in the delight of self-congratulation.

Self-examination has two primary purposes: recognition, confession and repentance of sin, and developing an ordering awareness of our own soul that helps organize our lives around God, resulting in loving him with everything we've got. Marjorie Thompson, in *Soul Feast*, suggests that self-examination takes place through both an examination of conscience and an examination of consciousness.[1]

Examination of Conscience and Confession

In the examination of conscience we search our hearts for sin for the purpose of confession and repentance. This is the practice encouraged in 1 Corinthians 11:27-29: "A man ought to examine himself before he eats of the bread and drinks of the cup." The thought of shining a light into the dark recesses of our soul can be intimidating and not particularly inviting. It is scary to be vulnerable and open, even within the secrecy of our own hearts. We'd much rather not think about our sins or confront our fears and frailties. But the exhortation to examination and confession is not for the purpose of punishment or naked exposure. It is an invitation to freedom. When Christ invites us to lay down our

Have mercy on me, O God,
according to your unfailing love;
according to your great compassion
blot out my transgressions.
Wash away all my iniquity
and cleanse me from my sin.
PSALM 51:1-2

burdens in exchange for his yoke, one of those burdens is our sins and failures. When we hold on to sin or ignore it we add weight to the heavy load that is crippling our walk. Our souls groan under the heaviness of this baggage we cling too. When we acknowledge and confess our sins we undo the straps binding us to these deadweights and we experience lightness and freedom and joy.

The initial opening up and shining of the light can be painful like any physical examination of an ailing part of our body. I injured my shoulder recently (not practicing yoga!) and I needed a thorough examination to determine the nature of the injury. It was a very painful process of probing and testing the joint, but very necessary and now the healing can begin with appropriate therapy and care. When we lay our sins before God and repent of them, the pain is temporary and the healing is promised. We do well to remember that we are not telling him anything he does not already know anyway! "For a man's ways are in full view of the LORD, and he examines all his paths" (Proverbs 5:21). When we open our hearts to His searching and confess our sin, "he does not treat us as our sins deserve or repay us according to our iniquities. For as high as the heavens are above the earth, so great is his love for those who fear him; as far as the east is from the west, so far has he removed our transgressions from us" (Psalm 103:10-12).

A model for our confession is found in Psalm 51. This is David's confession and cry to God for mercy after being confronted by the prophet Nathan for seducing Bathsheba and killing her husband to cover his sin. Our sins may pale in comparison to David's acts, or they may not. Either way we have the same call to repentance and the same hope and promise of mercy, forgiveness and redemption.

> Cleanse me with hyssop, and I will be clean;
> wash me, and I will be whiter than snow.

> Create in me a pure heart, O God,
> and renew a steadfast spirit within me.

> You do not delight in sacrifice, or I would bring it;
> you do not take pleasure in burnt offerings.
> The sacrifices of God are a broken spirit;
> a broken and contrite heart,
> O God, you will not despise (Psalm 51:7,10,16-17)

When we have examined our conscience and confessed our sin we need to believe God's promise that he is faithful and just and will forgive us our sin and purify us from all unrighteousness (1 John 1:9). We *are* washed and clean, he *has* blotted out all our transgressions and we stand whiter than snow. The weight has been lifted from our soul and we will find true peace. "In repentance and rest is your salvation, in quietness and trust is your strength" (Isaiah 30:15).

Examination of Consciousness

When you are on your beds, search
yourselves and be silent.
PSALM 4:4

Self-examination is not merely a penitential practice. We also want to carefully observe our actions and interactions, be mindful of where God's grace has intersected our lives, question our motives and consider our desires and disappointments. Marjorie Thompson tells us, "The examination of consciousness is a process of becoming aware of the contents of our consciousness, so that we can respond before God in an appropriate way. It is more concerned with the level of our awareness than with particular character flaws or behavioral lapses."[2] Our objective in the examination of our consciousness is to consider our day and how we lived it in the light of God's word, His grace and His love. Through this self-examination we seek to discern and to surrender to God's leading and direction. A helpful way to do this is to review the steps of the *Ignatian daily examen.*

Ignatius of Loyola, the founder of the Jesuit order in the 16th century, instituted the daily examen as part of his *Spiritual Exercises.* This daily exercise in self-examination has been practiced by Christians of both Catholic and Protestant persuasion for centuries and has been adapted by many different writers and church teachers as a model for self-examination. The examen has been called both an examination of conscience and consciousness, and while it does incorporate confession and repentance, it is a much broader exercise of self-awareness. Most often the method is recommended for use as a prayerful review at the end of your day. However it can be adapted to any time of day.

There are five basic steps to follow. These will vary slightly in how they are described and their order depending on what source you read. The Daily Examen included here is my paraphrase of the full version found on the *Finding God* website of the Loyola Press. [3]

The Daily Examen

1. Stillness: Recalling God's Presence

Choose a quiet place and posture of prayer. Resting pose at the end of yoga practice is ideal. Relax in God's presence and invite the Holy Spirit to help you honestly consider your day, your actions and responses in different situations. With the Spirit's guidance, recognize what draws you to God and what pulls you away from Him.

2. Gratitude: Expressing Thankfulness

Review your day and give thanks to God for his gifts. Try not to choose what to be thankful for but rather give thanks for what He brings to mind. Consider the physical blessings and the small graces of your day. Recall the gifts He has given you to share with others. Pause and express gratitude to God.

3. Reflection: Looking Back on Your Day

Review the day again and consider how you acted in the different situations you faced. Remember your feelings and motives to see if you followed God's will. Ask yourself when you were aware of God's presence. Did you have opportunities to grow in faith, hope, and love? Did you act with God's grace? By reflecting on how we did and didn't act we develop a greater sensitivity to acting with grace and following God's will.

4. Sorrow: Asking for Forgiveness

After recalling and reflecting on the actions of your day with the guidance of the Holy Spirit, spend time in conversation with God. Express sorrow for the times you failed to follow his direction and ask him to be with you the next time you are in a similar situation. Give thanks for the grace that enabled you to follow his will.

5. Hopefulness: Resolving to Grow

Ask God to help you as you look forward to a new day tomorrow. Resolve to cooperate and trust in the loving guidance of the Father, Son and the Holy Spirit. You may choose to conclude your time with God with the Lord's Prayer.

Ideally, we should be examining ourselves daily. If this is a new idea for you and you have never really taken time for self-examination you may want to start with a dedicated half-day or day for a life review and spiritual inventory. Going through a review like this can help you sort through all your "stuff" and give you a better grasp of the big picture of your life. This then helps guide your daily self-examination. There are many excellent materials available that can help guide you through this process. When we regularly take a personal inventory we keep the account short and regular self-examination should not take a very long time.

Self-examination is particularly well-suited to the quiet resting time at the beginning and end of each yoga class or private practice. You could start your yoga practice with an examination of conscience and prayer of confession. This is like starting with a clean slate, freeing you to spend the rest of the time in meaningful worship or listening and learning. Then, you could end the practice with examination of consciousness. From there you can proceed to the rest of your day with a clear conscience and purposefully be watching and listening for God's leading.

Socrates stated that the unexamined life is not worth living. I don't know if I would go that far but I would say that the examined life is better lived. If we are weighed down by unconfessed sin, living is hard. If we are foggy or unclear in our thinking and motives, we get distracted and life just happens and maybe not in the way we would like. It has been very popular to talk about Purpose in the last few years. When we take the time for self-examination and develop self-awareness, we can discern and live our purpose with greater intention. Housekeeping of our soul creates and maintains order so that it can be that organizing principle that orients our whole life around God and his purposes for us.

A YAHWEH YOGA STORY

Worshiping God through the practice of Yahweh Yoga has brought peace to my once stressed out lifestyle. Initially, my intention for beginning yoga was to heal a severe knee injury from training for a half-marathon. What I got in return was not only a healed knee but a healed life. Practicing yoga showed me that my knee injury was a symptom of a bigger problem of not taking proper care of myself on many levels. Yahweh Yoga has helped me to accept myself where I am and encouraged me to progress physically, emotionally and spiritually. Now I'm easier on myself and those around me.

In my last year of practicing at Yahweh Yoga, family members have noticed the positive changes in my personality. I have lost weight, become stronger, more fit, and closer to my Lord and Savior Jesus Christ. The Christian love shown at Yahweh Yoga has changed my life forever.
-Lisa

Silence and solitude. Meditation. Self-examination. These are disciplines of yoga and disciplines of the Christian life. All of these serve our quest to feed our hungry souls. When we look to God to satisfy our inner hunger and thirst, we will be filled.

He promises it.

We start out like David, with empty hands spread out before us, pleading for God. "I remember the days of long ago; I meditate on all your works and consider what your hands have done. I spread out my hands to you; my soul thirsts for you like a parched land" (Psalm 143:5-6).

Then our empty hands will be filled to overflowing, and out of our hearts will stream praises to God for his faithfulness. Being intentional about care for our soul will lead us to worship God, to loving him with our heart, soul, mind and strength.

> Let them give thanks to the LORD for his unfailing love
> and his wonderful deeds for men,
> for he satisfies the thirsty and fills
> the hungry with good things (Psalm 107:8-9).

[1] Marjorie J. Thompson, *Soul Feast: An Invitation to the Christian Spiritual Life,* (Louisville, Kent: Westminster John Knox Press, 2005), p.91.
[2] Thompson, *Soul Feast,* p.99.
[3] "Prayerfully Reviewing Your Day" *Prayer and Spirituality. Finding God* © 2007 Loyola Press. *www.findinggod.org/m_frmwork.asp?id=99764* (November 5, 2007).

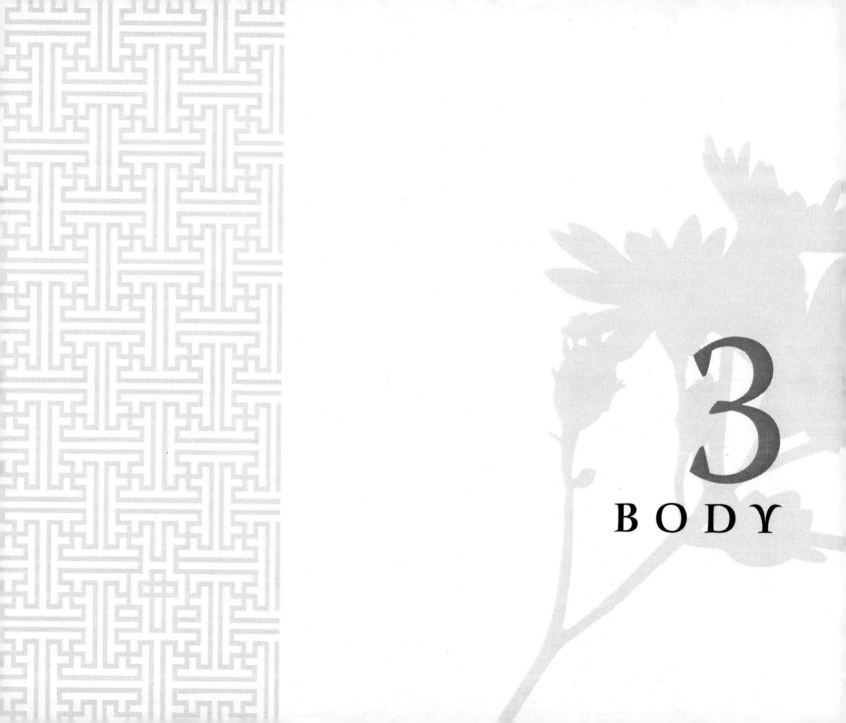

3

BODY

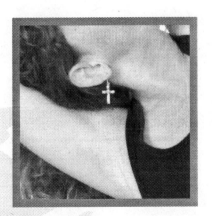 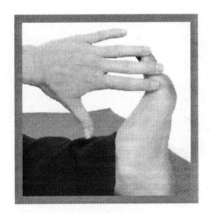 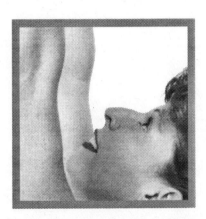

Do you not know that your body is
a temple of the holy spirit, who is in you,
whom you have received from God?
You are not your own; you were bought at a price.
Therefore, honor God with your body.
1 CORINTHIANS 6:19-20

CHAPTER EIGHT
Beautiful

HEALTH AND THE body are hot topics today. Headlines about obesity, cancer and environmental hazards compete with ads for miracle weight-loss plans, alternative therapies and organic lifestyles. There is always a new list of the Top Ten Miracle Foods that Prevent Cancer and Aging. I find myself trying to concoct an all-star healthy meal out of blueberries, salmon, artichokes, almonds and dark chocolate. Healthy? Yes. Tasty? Questionable.

We are more health conscious and body conscious than ever. It can be overwhelming to make sense of and apply the deluge of health information that we have at our fingertips. The fact is we are better informed than any previous generation about making healthy choices in our lifestyles. We know more about the importance of exercise, balanced diets and early detection of diseases than ever before. Transfats are evil, cholesterol is both good and bad, try for five servings of fruits and vegetables a day, watch your fiber intake, get regular exercise and enough sleep—we all know what we *should* do to guard and improve our physical health. But I suspect a majority of us (self included) are like Paul:

> I do not understand what I do. For what I want to do I do not do, but what I hate I do...I have the desire to do what is good but I cannot carry it out. For what I do is not the good I want to do; no; the evil I do not want to do—this I keep on doing! ...So I find this law at work. When I want to do good, evil is right there with me (Romans 7:15,18,19,21).

For you created my inmost being;
You knit me together in my
mother's womb.
I praise you because I am fearfully
and wonderfully made;
Your works are wonderful.
I know that full well.
PSALM 139:13-14

He has made everything beautiful in
its time.
ECCLESIASTES 3:11

I want to be good, I really do! Why can't I do it? I want to go to the gym but I take a detour through the drive-through on the way. I want to go for a daily walk but I turn on HGTV and sit down with a bag of potato chips. I buy oatmeal but I eat scrambled eggs and bacon. I put on my yoga DVD and I find that Ben & Jerry are right there with me!

Paul, of course, was speaking of our struggle with sin in general and our hope is in Christ's redeeming work in our lives. When we place our trust in Christ our hearts are transformed and our minds become renewable. Our frustrations and struggles to live a changed life come because we still wrestle with our untransformed bodies and their appetites. How do we win the battle? Earlier in Romans Paul said this:

> Do not let sin reign in your mortal body so that you obey its evil desires. Do not offer the parts of your body to sin as instruments of wickedness but rather offer yourselves to God, as those who have been brought from death to life; and offer the parts of your body as instruments of righteousness (Romans 6:12-13).

One of the first steps in overcoming the battle of the body is changing our perspective. We need to understand first that neglect and abuse of our bodies through unhealthy living is a sin.* What are the two biggest obstacles to health in our western society today?

---

* Again, I want to be careful to stress that we are not saying that sickness or poor health is necessarily evidence of sin or that God guarantees us health if we live a righteous life. That is a very destructive message of the Health and Wealth movement that has caused a lot of pain. There are many factors that influence our health over which we have no control. But there are other factors that we can control – our stewardship of our health rests on these.

Overeating or unhealthy eating and inactivity or lack of exercise. In biblical terms, gluttony and sloth. Proverbs warns us to put a knife to our throats if we are given to gluttony, and that the sluggard's craving will be the death of him. You will remember that God destroyed the cities of Sodom and Gomorrah for their sinful ways. Ezekiel tells us that "Sodom's sins were *pride, gluttony, and laziness*," and that these sins kept them from tending to the needy and poor. So God wiped them out.[1]

God takes these things very seriously. We discussed earlier that the goal in caring for ourselves is ultimately to better love and serve God and others. Gluttony and laziness are significant obstacles to that goal. We started our journey in self-care with paying attention to the needs of our soul, spending time in God's presence and listening to him, exchanging our ways for his ways, our thoughts for his thoughts. When we do this our perspective changes. With God's eyes we will see the need for care of our body differently and take to heart the warnings against gluttony and sloth. This is the beginning of not letting our appetites rule us.

With God's perspective then, we make a choice about what to do with our bodies. We do not have to be slaves to our cravings. Instead we offer our bodies to God as instruments of righteousness. This means we use them for Him; we serve Him. And everything we do with and to our bodies is then judged against God's standard. Am I serving him in righteousness? Will this decision help me to do that better or hurt my ability to serve? "Do you not know that your body is a temple of the Holy Spirit, who is in you, whom you have received from God? You are not your own; you were bought at a price. **Therefore honor God with your body**" (1 Corinthians 6:19-20, emphasis added).

Paul urges us to offer our bodies as "living sacrifices, holy and pleasing to God" and tells us this is one way we worship Him. *The Message* paraphrase of this verse puts it beautifully into today's language:

> Take your everyday, ordinary life—your sleeping, eating, going-to-work, and walking-around life—and place it before God as an offering. Embracing what God does for you is the best thing you can do for him (Romans 12:1).

Caring for our bodies and serving God with them honors God! When we honor God with our bodies, we are honoring him as our Creator, Redeemer and Sustainer in whom we live, move and have our being.

God's Amazing Design

Our bodies are an incredible gift from God and a testimony to his genius as Creator and Designer. In His infinite wisdom, God created our bodies and designed all their intricate systems and how these systems work together for life. When we engage in practices that support and optimize the systems of our bodies we acknowledge and honor God's design. When we abuse or neglect our bodies, taxing and stressing those systems, we dishonor

CHRISTIAN YOGA ✠ Beautiful

God's creation. Dr. Richard Swenson has written extensively about the marvelous precision and intricacy of our bodies in his book *More than Meets the Eye*. Here are just a few facts to ponder:

- We have sixty thousand miles of blood vessels in our bodies.

- We manufacture over two million red blood cells a second.

- The hemoglobin in each red blood cell can carry a million oxygen molecules to our cells.

- Our ears can distinguish between two thousand different pitches.

- Our nose can tell the difference between ten thousand different smells.

- In one third of a second our retina can solve nonlinear differential equations that would take a supercomputer 100 years to solve.

- Our brain can hold information equivalent to twenty-five million books.

- We hold in our brain three trillion pictures.[2]

And we can laugh, we can cry, we can create, we can dance, we can sing, we can love and our hearts can be broken. We are truly God's beautiful masterpieces. We *are* fearfully and wonderfully made.

shoulders were stiff and sore. Two days after I left the hospital, I went to a restorative class at Yahweh Yoga where the focus is on slow, gentle movements. I propped myself up on bolsters and blankets and lay with my arms outstretched. Because the movement was slow, I could gradually increase the stretch at my own pace. Some of the class was more than I could handle but by the end I felt like a new woman. My posture improved, I felt stronger and my mood was considerably better.

Throughout the next weeks of my recovery I continued to attend yoga class. Most of my physical milestones occurred there, where I was able to very slowly coax my body to the next step. Most of all, I was able to embrace the slow. With yoga, I was familiar with my body and it's need to recover. I didn't need to push it beyond what it was ready for. I recognized the importance of rest and I valued it. Yoga was a key factor in my recovery physically and emotionally. Five weeks after open heart surgery I was able to travel to the Middle East to teach at a women's conference. Something I believe was only possible because of the grace of God in my very deliberate, slow recovery.

—Kelli

Beautiful in God's Eyes

I realize we may not always feel like we are a masterpiece. Sometimes I look in the mirror and what I see is merely fearful, not fearfully and wonderfully made. At those times I have to ask whose standard I am measuring myself against. The world's or God's? His standard or mine? God's definition of beauty is very different than the world's. True beauty comes from within. "Charm is deceptive and beauty is fleeting but a woman who fears the Lord is to be praised"(Proverbs 31:30). There is a lot of pressure on us today to be a certain size and to look a certain way and it is hard. I know. I am a size twelve woman in a size two world and I'm never going to be a size two. But God doesn't want me to be a size two. He wants me to find my identity in him, not the number on my waistband.

Did you know that God takes delight in his children? Do you consider yourself delightful? Psalm 18:19 says, "he rescued me because he delighted in me." He delights in us the way he made us. The Bible describes God as the Potter and us as the clay he shapes into pots, as he sees fit. Paul asked the question, "Shall the pot say to the potter, 'why did you make me like this?'" No. Big pots, little pots, grand pots, humble pots, cracked and wobbly pots—we are all masterpieces made for His glory and he has made everything beautiful in its time. We can all be beautiful pots that glorify God and radiate his love.

Body and Spirituality

Somewhere along the way we have lost a clear idea about where our body fits into our spirituality. Physical health has been relegated to the secular domain. A common question and complaint against Christian yoga is this: "Why should we exercise in church? You can go to the gym for that." I ask back, why shouldn't care for our bodies happen in a sacred setting? Why shouldn't we promote physical health at church? Not necessarily in our weekly worship services but surely in our midweek programs. I am not sure there is a compelling reason to identify the pursuit of physical health as a wholly secular practice.

For many of us our church experience both on Sundays and in midweek programs is all about head and heart but not body. We sing enthusiastically about lifting our hands up to God with them firmly in our pockets. We sing about falling down and laying our crowns while sitting cross-legged. We raise an eyebrow at the swaying hip or waving hand, and we're not sure what to do with someone who sits instead of stands or stands instead of sits. If this is not your experience be so grateful!

I confess I am very inhibited about my body in worship and I am fully aware of the irony. There are times I long to raise my hands in worship but I feel so self-conscious about it that I don't. My inhibition comes only from myself not my church. My experience with Christian yoga changed that for me and introduced me to a whole new dimension of worship. Christian yoga can help us understand how our body fits with our spirituality.

Engaging our body in our spirituality greatly enriches and expands our experience. To me this is very similar to the theories of learning styles. We all have different ways that we best absorb, process and express information. We may be strongly visual, auditory or kinesthetic (movement and touch oriented). When we use all our senses in our learning we learn better. Being mindful of how we learn best helps us to engage in a way that is most meaningful and effective. I have a child who needs to experience his environment, not just observe it. He has to jump through space, roll on the floor, flip over the couch, touch his brother and find all forty ways to sit on a chair. He is a kinesthetic learner who more readily absorbs teaching when his body is engaged, moving and touching.

So will we more readily absorb truth, hide God's word in our heart more deeply and feel His presence more keenly when we engage our bodies and all our senses. Moving our bodies in worship, or participating in symbolic ritual like communion or washing feet, helps move our head knowledge into heart wisdom. This also moves us further in our desire to live out the greatest commandment to love the Lord with all our heart, soul, mind and strength.

Christian yoga helped me to understand this in such a concrete way. When I first started practicing I had to concentrate so much on what my body was doing that I did not have much of a spiritual experience. You may find the same thing but persevere! With regular practice I became familiar with the postures and flows and could move without requiring too much concentration. Then the beautiful worship music and gentle leading words of the instructor moved me into worship and contemplation. In spite of myself, I found my hands were raised to God! While standing in Mountain or Warrior my hands were raised as part of the posture at the same time that my heart was moved in praise. With my body and my heart united in an expression of worship I experienced something so much deeper of God. Now, granted, I can do the same thing in church. But in yoga class my whole body is being moved and I feel a freedom from inhibition. No one is watching me there. I haven't reached that freedom in church yet, but someday I will.

Sometimes the posture of my heart leads the posture of my body—my body responds to what my heart is feeling or my mind is thinking. I may find I want to lay down flat out in a position of submission and confession before God. In a time of great need I hold out my empty hands asking for his mercy and provision. In these times my body is following my heart.

Sometimes, however, I need the posture of my body to lead my heart. I think of Job. Everything he owned and everyone he loved was destroyed. He ripped his robes and shaved his head but instead of cursing, he fell before the Lord in worship. *The Lord gives and the Lord takes away, praise the name of the Lord.* I don't think Job felt like worshiping God right then, but he chose to and he did so with his body. There are times we do not feel like worshiping or we do not want to confess. Sometimes we'd rather hold onto our sin or our pain and nurse it. In these times we have to make a choice and we can use our bodies to help us do that. We can make that choice by raising our hands, bowing in confession, falling prostrate, by leading with our bodies. Our hearts and minds will follow.

Discipline or Asceticism?

In a discussion of body and spirituality we must address the difference between discipline and asceticism. The word asceticism came from the Greek and originally meant "exercise or training." It has since evolved to refer to extreme or severe self-denial and self-mortification through renunciation of worldly pleasures and comforts. Both Christianity and Hinduism have strong histories of asceticism. There are all kinds of bizarre practices of devotion or *tapas* that one can find in Hinduism. In general these are very physically punishing vows. Standing *babas* vow never to sit, even in sleep, and spend their entire lives in swings or slings. Their feet become deformed and severely damaged. Extreme fasting, standing in freezing water or under the scorching sun without shelter are some other examples. The Hindu hopes to accomplish purification, atone for past sins, find a shortcut through their karma or attain spiritual growth through such punishment of the self.

Some of these vows are similar to displays of Christian asceticism in church history, which were equally bizarre. Some early desert fathers and hermits made vows to live in caves with only bread and water or to live on small platforms at the top of towers for decades. Similarly they sought penance for their sins and a deeper expression of piety. Today there are still some church-based orders of Flagellants, people who whip and torture themselves to being bloody as part of the season of Lent, even culminating in self-crucifixion. This is not how God intended we treat our bodies.

The apostle Paul spoke out against such excessive asceticism in Colossians 2:23: "Such regulations indeed have an appearance of wisdom, with their self-imposed worship, their false humility and their harsh treatment of the body, but they lack any value in restraining sensual indulgence." Richard Foster writes that asceticism makes an unbiblical division between a good spiritual world and an evil material world and so finds salvation in paying as little attention as possible to the physical realm.[3] There is no freedom in asceticism.

Instead of a severe asceticism we have pictures of self-discipline and self-control in the Bible. In this context *discipline* recaptures the original meaning of asceticism: to train or to exercise. In Christian yoga we are not seeking an asceticism of the body but rather a training and exercising of it. We don't hold uncomfortable postures for unreasonable amounts of time to punish our flesh or escape from it. We may make choices of abstinence but we do this for the health of our body not the punishing of it. We also make these choices of discipline in the context of freedom and as a means of freedom from the tyranny of man's rules and the rule of sin. Ultimately, we are caring for our bodies and exercising as only one part of training ourselves for godliness.

Discipline yourself for the purpose of godliness; for bodily discipline is only of little profit, but godliness is profitable for all things, since it holds promise for the present life and also for the life to come (1 Timothy 4:7-9 NASB).

You've all been to the stadium and seen the athletes race. Everyone runs; one wins. Run to win. All good athletes train hard. They do it for a gold medal that tarnishes and fades. You're after one that's gold eternally. I don't know about you, but I'm running hard for the finish line. I'm giving it everything I've got. No sloppy living for me! I'm staying alert and in top condition. I'm not going to get caught napping, telling everyone else all about it and then missing out myself (1 Corinthians 9:24-27 *The Message*).

We're training to run the race and to finish it well, with our eyes fixed on the author and perfecter of our faith, Jesus.

Self-Care for the Body

Caring for our bodies does not have to be a complicated endeavor. If we pay attention to a few simple things we will start to reap health benefits very quickly.

1. *Nutrition.* It is very important to be mindful about what we put into our bodies. Make an effort to eat whole, unprocessed foods and choose organic where possible. Aim for a

balanced diet with lots of variety. Quality foods are the building blocks for healthy bodies.

2. *Rest.* We are chronically sleep deprived and unfortunately, sleep deficits are accumulative. Getting enough rest is foundational to good health. God established a beautiful and necessary rhythm of work and rest when he instituted the Sabbath. Enjoy rest as a reward for your work – you will be honoring God and your body.

3. *Exercise.* Regular exercise is vital. If we live sedentary lives our bodies and their systems atrophy. Exercise contributes to our physical, mental and emotional well-being. Numerous studies are demonstrating that exercise does not have to be excessively intense or extended to be beneficial but it does need to be regular. Moderate physical activity several times a week will achieve results.

4. *Stress Reduction.* Stress is the culprit in so many of our disorders of both body and soul. Reducing stress factors can change your outlook and your health. Often there are simple changes that you can make to lower your stress levels. Radical lifestyle changes are sometimes necessary but worth it.

There are many resources available today to help you pursue a healthier lifestyle. Christian yoga will help you directly address your needs for exercise and stress reduction. In the next chapter you will read about the many health benefits that come with the regular practice of Christian yoga. As you practice Christian yoga you will discover how it also helps you to develop healthy perspectives and priorities for nutrition and rest. As we start to see our bodies and our health through God's eyes we will be encouraged in our stewardship of them.

Your body is an amazing and beautiful gift from God, a miracle and masterpiece of design beyond our comprehension. Dr. Swenson invites us to "never presume to fully understand it—physically, spiritually or ecclesiastically. Instead stand in awe of God who can package atoms in such a mystical, glorious form."[4]

Let's live like we are glorious masterpieces. Let's honor God by looking after our bodies with the same respect and care we would use to look after a great work of art—because that is what we are.

---

[1] Ezekiel 16:49-50 NLT, emphasis added.
[2] Richard A. Swenson, *More than Meets the Eye: Fascinating Glimpses of God's Power and Design,* (Colorado Springs: NavPress, 2000), selected facts from chapters 1-7.
[3] Richard Foster, *Celebration of Discipline*, p.84.
[4] Richard Swenson, *More than Meets the Eye*, p.100.

CHAPTER NINE

Benefits of Yoga

AS YOGA HAS grown in popularity more and more research has been done investigating the health benefits of the practice. Clear evidence has been found that yoga is very beneficial for physical health and yoga has entered mainstream healthcare as a therapy for various ailments. It is being used in major cardiac and health centers throughout the nation as a therapy for recovery and rehabilitation. Yoga has also been recognized as especially restorative for those suffering with arthritis and other degenerative diseases. Chances are you are picking up this book because you have had yoga prescribed to you by your healthcare provider.

Yoga postures also closely parallel physical therapy protocols particularly for back and hip pain. I have been to physical therapy many times for problems with my lower back that started with an injury in my late teens. When I started attending yoga classes I was pleasantly surprised by how many of the postures were very similar, if not identical, to the physical therapy exercises I was supposed to be doing for my back. But yoga was far more enjoyable and cheaper and easier to practice regularly. Yoga is actually the first physical exercise regimen that I have successfully followed for an extended time in almost twenty years of dealing with a herniated disk and, more recently, arthritis in my back. Through regular yoga practice I have also enjoyed significant and sustained relief from the chronic pain that comes with disc problems. When I don't keep up with regular practice I feel it! I am so motivated to get back to it because pain is not worth it.

Dear friend, I pray that you may enjoy good health and that all may go well with you, even as your soul is getting along well.
3 JOHN 2

SKELETAL & MUSCULAR SYSTEMS
- Arthritis
- Osteoporosis
- Back Pain
- Knee pain
- Plantar Fascitis
- Kyphosis (rounding of upper spine)
- Scoliosis
- Sciatica

CARDIOVASCULAR SYSTEM
- Hypertension
- Heart Disease
- Angina

GASTROINTESTINAL SYSTEM
- Irritable Bowel Syndrome
- Constipation
- Heartburn

NERVOUS SYSTEM
- Depression
- Anxiety
- Migraines

RESPIRATORY SYSTEM
- Asthma
- Bronchitis
- Allergies

Benefits for the Body

The practice of yoga is beneficial for all the major systems of the body, supporting their normal function and aiding in the relief of diseases and rehabilitation from injury. Some of the systems are noted in the sidebar with just a few of the ailments that are improved with regular yoga practice. Some of the observed general health benefits of a regular yoga practice are:

- Pulse rate decreases
- Respiratory rate decreases
- Blood pressure decreases
- Cardiovascular efficiency increases
- Respiratory efficiency increases
- Gastrointestinal function normalizes
- Endocrine function normalizes
- Excretory functions improve
- Anxiety and depression decrease
- Grip strength increases
- Eye-hand coordination improves
- Mood improves
- Integrated functioning of body parts improves

- Dexterity skills improve
- Reaction time improves
- Posture improves
- Increased muscle tone
- Endurance increases
- Energy levels increase
- Weight normalizes
- Sleep improves
- Steadiness and balance improve
- Pain decreases
- Immunity increases
- Memory and concentration improves
- Increased flexibility and range of motion in joints[1]

Yoga includes weight bearing exercise, stretching, and higher intensity practices offer cardiovascular benefits—all the forms of exercise most commonly recommended for general health. Instead of trying to find time for all these different types of exercise, you can set aside time for an hour of yoga several times a week and enjoy all these benefits from one practice. Yoga is also a proven stress reliever. Over the past couple of decades medical research has clearly proven links between the body's response to stress and illness and disease. Health can easily be improved by effectively dealing with stress.

Yoga is not an attempt to hide a religious agenda in an apparently healthy system in order to take advantage of the growing health consciousness of society today. It IS one of the healthiest and most beneficial health practices available that also easily accommodates disability, injury, disease, obesity, and age limitations. Christians should be able to enjoy and benefit from the physical health available through the regular practice of yoga.

There is a universal condition of humanity that transcends race, religion and culture— we all have bodies! And we all have souls and hearts that are the center of our being. Our bodies and our souls share a common experience of health and pain and disease. We all suffer with aches and pains and disorders. Cancer has the same effects for an American, a Canadian and an African. Arthritis affects a Christian the same way it affects a Hindu or Buddhist. The drugs, treatments and therapies for diseases and disabilities likewise do not discriminate.

As Christians we don't dismiss medical advances and treatments because they weren't developed by Christian scientists and doctors. We don't say, "I'm sorry doctor, I can't take that high blood pressure medication because it was not developed in the church." That would be a rather medieval approach to health and not terribly effective. In the same way, neither should we be dismissive of the health benefits of yoga because it has come to us through a different system of belief.

Benefits for the Soul

One of the reasons yoga is so healthy for us is that it addresses the whole person. So many of our sicknesses today are linked to stress. We have yet to fully understand how emotional and spiritual distress manifest in physical distress but it is being observed and documented all the time. The Bible tells us the same truth:

> I am bowed down and brought very low;
> all day long I go about mourning.
> My back is filled with searing pain;
> there is no health in my body.
> I am feeble and utterly crushed;
> I groan in anguish of heart.
> All my longings lie open before you, O Lord;

my sighing is not hidden from you.

My heart pounds, my strength fails me;

even the light has gone from my eyes (Psalm 38:6-10).

Be merciful to me, O LORD, for I am in distress;

my eyes grow weak with sorrow,

my soul and my body with grief.

My life is consumed by anguish

and my years by groaning;

my strength fails because of my affliction,

and my bones grow weak (Psalm 31:9-10).

In both of these Psalms we see a picture of David in mental and emotional anguish; his soul is in distress and his body is falling apart because of it. I know each one of us can relate to that kind of anguish. But God is merciful and answers our cries of distress. "But I call to God, and the LORD saves me. Evening, morning and noon I cry out in distress, and he hears my voice"(Psalm 55:16-17). "I will be glad and rejoice in your love, for you saw my affliction and knew the anguish of my soul. You have not handed me over to the enemy but have set my feet in a spacious place" (Psalm 31:7-8).

that I was able to experience.

Directing four PT clinics and raising two children keeps me busy but I find the practice of yoga has allowed me to focus on my health, flexibility and strength as well as the additional benefits of stress relief. No two yoga classes are the same but no matter how you are feeling you can adapt the class to meet your needs.

In addition, I am practicing yoga as "age prevention" for the three things that are profoundly reduced during the natural aging process: flexibility, strength and balance. All three of these areas are addressed in yoga practice and with regular work you will see measurable and significant results. It is astounding that at the ripe old age of forty I was able to make such gains in all areas. I am delighted to be able to enjoy hiking, skiing and running without pain or fatigue.

—Maria, PT

Inextricably tied up with our physical health is the health of our soul. We can lay the anguish of our souls before God and ask him for healing that will bring health to our bones and our hearts. "He heals the brokenhearted and binds up their wounds" (Psalm 147:3).

When our yoga studio describes itself as "An Oasis for Self-Care", we think of that "spacious place" in Psalm 31. It has been especially rewarding over the last few years to watch women and men who are in a lot of soul-pain come to yoga class and find healing through time with God. When we take the time through Christian yoga to tend to our soul at the same time as tending to our bodies we will reap wonderful health benefits. We will "enjoy good health…even as our souls are getting along well."

---

[1]"Health Benefits of Yoga - Why Yoga Exercise is Good for You," *www.abc-of-yoga.com/beginnersguide/yogabenefits.asp* (November 6, 2007)

CHAPTER TEN
Breathe

BREATH IS LIFE. We take our first breath and breathe our last at the opening and closing moments of our brief span on earth. Each breath in between is a reminder that our life is a gift from God. How odd it is that in times of pressure and stress we often forget to breathe. We gasp for air both literally and figuratively. We need the breath of God to support our wheezing attempts to soldier on through these times. We also need to actually breathe air deep into our lungs. Purposeful and mindful breathing energizes our bodies and enables us to function so much more effectively. The breath is foundational to Christian yoga practice.

O Lord, you are the God who gives breath to all creatures.
NUMBERS 27:16

Breathe on me, breath of God.
EDWIN HATCH

Physiology of Breathing

Breathing supplies our bodies with the oxygen vital for our survival. Oxygen is necessary for the combustion of energy in our cells. When we breathe, air fills our lungs and oxygen molecules are picked up by the blood and carried to each of our cells. The red blood cells deliver oxygen and pick up carbon dioxide, a waste product of cellular combustion, which is then carried back to the lungs and breathed out. When you inhale your diaphragm goes down as air rushes into your lungs. The action of the diaphragm widens your rib cage and also pushes your abdomen down and forward. When you exhale your diaphragm returns to its original position, as air releases from your lungs. Your abdomen goes in and up when you breathe out.

A large majority of people are chest breathers. This means that they breathe shallowly, using primarily their chest muscles instead of their abdominal muscles. Most of the air exchange then occurs at the top of the lung tissues. The bottom third of the lung is left unused but this is where most of the blood flow takes place in the lungs. Chest breathing is very inefficient for the necessary exchange of oxygen and carbon dioxide. By making a conscious effort to breathe more deeply and fully, using more of the abdominal muscles you can start to reverse the inefficient habits of chest breathing. Proper breathing strengthens the immune system, can increase your metabolism and help modify your blood pressure. It can also increase your lung capacity overall.

Most of us don't think about our breathing too often. Breathing is one of our body's autonomic functions, which means we don't have to consciously make an effort to breathe. It just happens, in the same way our heart beats without our having to think about it. Breathing is different from other autonomic functions however in that we can take control over our breath—like an override function. This override ability is self-protecting just like an override on machinery is a safety feature. If our oxygen supply is threatened by water or noxious gases we can hold our breath. If our muscles demand extra oxygen because of heavy exertion or sudden stress we can breath more deeply to increase the supply. We can hold our breath, change the pace and intensity, and change the depth of our breathing. Breathing also influences our emotional equilibrium.

Controlling our breath through intentional or purposeful breathing can increase our concentration, be relaxing or energizing and help us release stress. It also helps strengthen the connection between our bodies and our minds. Some of us are naturally comfortable in and with our bodies. Movement and coordination are easy, second-nature and graceful. Dancers and athletes often exhibit this natural grace. And then there are the rest of us who are not so at home in our own skin. Maybe you are like me—rhythmically challenged and left-right disabled. I have to really concentrate to clap on beat and I have to think carefully about moving my left or my right limbs into position. For people like us intentional and focused breathing helps build a stronger body-mind connection, allowing us to move more purposefully and perhaps even more gracefully.

Breathing Techniques

In yoga there are many breathing techniques that accomplish different things like relaxing or energizing or improving our focus. We are highlighting the most important and helpful techniques here. Always clear your nose prior to using any of these techniques and practice in room temperature or warmer.

Breath of De-Stress

Deep breathing in through the nose and out through the mouth affects your whole body. Full, deep breathing in through the nose and out through the mouth helps reduce tension and stress. More oxygen moves to the brain which helps relieve anxiety and calm the nervous system. The workload for the heart is reduced and the lungs grow more powerful and healthy. Breathing like this also eliminates toxins aiding digestion and enhancing the skin. Moving the diaphragm with deep breathing exercises massages abdominal organs, the stomach, small intestines, pancreas and the heart and helps blood to circulate more efficiently.

1. Be seated comfortably or lay flat on your back in a relaxed position.

2. Breathe very deeply in through the nose, feeling the air rush past the back of your throat.

3. Slowly exhale through the mouth with a quiet whooshing sound until the lungs are empty.

Caution: Some people get a little dizzy the first few times they try deep breathing of any kind. If you become lightheaded, slow your breathing and sit for a moment.

Abdominal Breath or the Natural Breath

This breath focuses on breathing deeply into the lungs, using the diaphragm and the abdomen. It begins to reset our patterns from shallow chest breathing to deep, healthy, belly breathing.

1. Lying down, place one hand on the belly and one hand on the heart.

2. Inhale deeply through the nose, while visualizing the lungs filling up with air all the way to the top.

3. Exhale slowly through the nose and picture the lungs completely emptying.

4. Feel the belly rise and fall with each inhale and exhale.

Three-part Breath or Complete Breath

The complete breath takes abdominal breathing further, expanding and stretching the lungs gently and increasing lung capacity. You start with filling the lower part of the lungs first, then you fill the middle and upper part. When exhaling you first empty the upper part of the lungs, then the middle, and last of all the lower part. Picture an empty vase. On the inhale, picture the vase filling from the bottom to the top with water. On the exhale, picture the vase emptying from the top to the bottom.

1. As you inhale, expand the abdomen first, then the ribs and then the chest. Inhale for a count of five.

2. As you exhale, retract the chest, then the ribs and then contract your abdomen, pulling it in toward your spine and pushing all the air out. Exhale for a count of 5.

3. Pause briefly and repeat.

Victorious or Ocean Sounding Breath

In Kids Yoga we call this the Darth Vader Breath. The sound created by this breath is like a soft hissing sound or a gentle snore. This is one of the most important breathing techniques in yoga. It increases body heat, calms and focuses the mind using gentle sound and helps you to relax more deeply. This breath can be used in a gentle, meditative way or in a forceful, energizing way. It will either lower or raise your blood pressure and heart rate accordingly. The Victorious Breath is helpful for pain reduction, insomnia, and migraines. The mouth stays shut for this breath.

1. Inhale through the nose for a count of five.

2. Exhale through the nose for a count of five. On the exhale you are constricting the back of the throat in order to have that ocean sound expelling from the nostrils. Really push the air completely out.

Alternate Nostril Breathing

This breath helps bring balance between your sympathetic (active) nervous system and your parasympathetic (relaxing) nervous system.

1. Be seated comfortably.

2. Place the right hand in front of the face. The thumb is placed by the right nostril. The pointer and center finger are placed between the eye brows. The ring and pinky finger are placed by the left nostril.

3. Close off the right nostril with the thumb.

4. Inhale deeply through the left nostril and then close it off with the pinky and ring finger.

5. Open and exhale through the right nostril.

6. Keep the right nostril open and inhale. Close it off then release the air out the left side. Continue for 10 breaths.

If you feel light headed please stop and breathe normally.

Breath of Fire or Bellows Breathing

This exercise strengthens the chest and diaphragm, loosens the spine, stretches the lungs and controls the breath at a different level. This is a very energizing breath and can be used as a quick pick-me-up any time you are feeling a lull in body energy. It is best not to practice this breath near bedtime.

1. Stand in mountain posture with your hands at your side.

2. On the inhale lift straight arms 15 inches, then immediately inhale again and lift arms another 15 inches. One more inhale and the arms come over the head.

3. Give a BIG loud exhale through the mouth as you bend the knees and reach down for the earth.

4. Repeat five times.

Breathe on Me, Breath of God

When God created Adam, he formed him from the earth and then *breathed* into him the breath of life and he became a "living being". How awesome that God breathes the breath of life into us. In the same way that we hunger and thirst for God, we breathe him too. He is our life. A popular worship song declares to God, "You are the air I breathe." Job cried out, "As long as I have life within me, the breath of God in my nostrils...."

As we learn to breathe more purposefully, more effectively, let's be mindful that it is God's breath in our nostrils. Let's thank him every day for our breath.

I bless God every chance I get;
my lungs expand with his praise.
I live and breathe God (Psalm 34:1-2 *The Message*).

CHAPTER ELEVEN
Begin

NOW IT IS time to get started with your Christian yoga practice! There are a few simple things you need to keep in mind in getting ready.

When

One of the beautiful gifts of yoga is you can practice anytime and almost anywhere. Yoga can be an energizing way to start your day or a relaxing way to end it. If you practice in the evening make sure you do not do any energizing postures such as headstands. These will interfere with your sleep. You will need to organize your yoga practice around when you eat however. It is best not to have eaten for an hour or two prior to practicing. Practice as often as you can; we recommend you practice for one hour three times per week at a minimum for optimum health. However, any time will still be beneficial. You can gradually work into a regular schedule.

Where

A structured yoga class can provide an environment that is most conducive for practice. The temperature can be regulated. The lighting can really set the mood. Some studios provide aromatherapy. A studio also provides some pampering items you may not have at your own home. Eye bags, bolsters, blankets, blocks and straps are often offered for your convenience. You will also find fellowship and community at a studio even though

Strengthen the feeble hands, steady the knees that give way; say to those with fearful hearts, "Be strong, do not fear; your God will come... he will come to save you."
ISAIAH 35:3-4

He gives strength to the weary and increases the power of the weak. Even youths grow tired and weary, and young men stumble and fall; but those who hope in the LORD will renew their strength. They will soar on wings like eagles; they will run and not grow weary, they will walk and not be faint.
ISAIAH 40:29-31

yoga is a primarily solitary practice. Solitude in the context of a like-minded community is a beautiful thing.

A home practice can be quite intimate for you and the Lord. Sometimes a DVD and a hour is the only time you can grab. Take advantage of a clear and clean space where you can do your postures. Make sure distractions can be eliminated before you begin.

The most important consideration in choosing a class or a DVD for your home practice is that you choose a place or materials that are God honoring and Christ centered. If there is not a Christian yoga class in your area, there may be some yoga classes that you can find at a local gym or YMCA that are very neutral in their spiritual emphasis. Pray for wisdom and evaluate the class in light of what we have discussed in this book. If you feel any hesitation or are uncomfortable with an instructor, trust that this is God leading you not to participate in this class.

Our wish would be for every city to have a Christian yoga studio like ours. In the meantime, Yahweh Yoga offers DVDs of all our classes that you can use in your home practice. Make sure you choose a DVD and class that is the appropriate level for you. Always start at the beginning and work up to intermediate and advanced levels gradually and carefully. There is no hurry.

Water

Drink plenty of water to keep hydrated. You need a minimum eight to twelve cups of water per day and even more to replace the fluid you lose during exercise. Depending on your size and perspiration rate, you lose about four cups of water per hour of exercise. There are lots of good reasons to make sure you are drinking enough water:

- Your body is 85% liquid.
- You lose about a quart a day just by breathing.
- Pure water flushes waste from the body.
- Builds muscle.
- Improves digestion.
- Helps with weight loss.
- Regulates body temperature.
- Lubricates the joints.
- Moisturizes and clears skin of blemishes.

You will want to keep a bottle of water handy for before, during and after practice.

Clothing

It is important to wear comfortable clothes that you can move in and that will move with you. It is not a good idea to wear anything too large or loose — you want your clothes to stay on your body in the postures including inversions (head lower than the heart.) Also, please be mindful of modesty in class. Pants or capris would be better than athletic shorts.

Equipment

A yoga mat is the only piece of "equipment" that you really need. These are made from "sticky" material which helps keep your hands and feet from slipping. This is very important for your safety. You can practice without a mat but it is risky and not preferable. As you spend more and more time on your mat it becomes a very sacred space for you — a place dedicated to prayer and your self-care. Be sure to choose a color that is soothing to you. Make sure the quality of the sticky mat is good. There are mats in every price range from $15.00 to $100.00. You may want to have a towel with you. It can be helpful for wiping sweat off your face, placing between the mat and your face, or folded as extra support for your knees or neck.

Yoga blocks, chairs, blankets, belts and bolsters are wonderful props or aids. If you do not have them at your home use a tie or long scarf for a belt. A block could be one of your favorite thick books. We all have a chair and a blanket right? This is why you can practice yoga anywhere. If you are restricted in your ability to get up and down off the floor or need to accommodate weak wrists or knees, many of the postures can be adapted using a chair. Yoga blocks can be used to support your hands when you cannot reach all the way to the floor to support yourself. Belts help you stretch when your hands cannot reach your toes.

Music

Music is a very important part of your Christian yoga practice. Soothing instrumental worship music will help you set your intention and focus your mind on your time with God. Of course, your personal taste will direct your music selection. In general, gentle and quiet music will be the most helpful in creating a time of solitude and sanctuary for meeting God. Music in a class should be organized in a way that follows the progression of the practice, starting gentle and restful, building in intensity and returning to calm and soothing.

If you are practicing at home, start with reading a passage from the Bible. You may also want to keep a journal handy to record anything after practice God teaches you or speaks to you about through your time of meditation with him.

Special Considerations

As with any new exercise regime, check with your doctor if you have any medical concerns or have not been active. Please pay careful attention to the notes for each posture. Headstands and Crow are for advanced practitioners. **Please do not attempt these until you have visited with a CYT or RYT/ E-RYT to learn the proper alignment**

first. Be very cautious about any contraindications that apply to you (bad knees, pregnancy, back sensitivity etc.)

These are some general precautions to keep in mind:

Pregnancy

Regular yoga practice during your pregnancy can be very beneficial and soothing but be aware that certain postures should be avoided such as those that involve laying on the back or belly. Also avoid any breath retentions. Get a video or book that is specifically designed for expectant mothers or attend a prenatal yoga class. These videos, books, and classes will cover postures that help to reduce back pain, swelling in the lower extremities, and misalignments due to weight changes. Many postures, like squats, will help prepare for natural childbirth and may help ease labor and delivery. During pregnancy, hormones cause joints in the body to become loose. Yoga postures can help to stabilize and strengthen these joints and promote flexibility in the muscles and fascia.

Glaucoma, other eye problems, and ear congestion

If you are experiencing problems with your eyes or ears, do not take your head below the level of your heart. Modifications would be hands on thighs for down dog and no inversions. Avoid breath retention.

Hypertension/High blood pressure

If you have high blood pressure and are on medication you should be just fine. **If you are NOT taking medication do NOT take your head below your heart.** Avoid breath retention.

Sciatica

Back bends are your friend...forward bends are not.

Menstruation

Some advise not to practice while menstruating and some say it is the best thing for you at this time. It is up to the individual. Every woman knows what feels good to their body and what is uncomfortable. Our advice is, if it is uncomfortable, stop. There is some concern that inversions like shoulder stands and headstands may cause retrograde flow so you will want to avoid these while actually menstruating. Many of the postures are excellent for bringing relief from PMS symptoms like anxiety, cramping and irritability.

How to proceed through yoga practice

Warm Up

Assume that the body is cold and stiff at the beginning of any practice. Picture in your mind a piece of taffy that has come out of the refrigerator. Imagine trying to stretch and pull it. Then imagine holding it in your hands for a few moments, warming it. Then pull it and stretch it. That is how we want to take care of our muscles and connective tissues. If we don't warm them first we risk injury. Always begin with a gentle and comforting warm up sequence. Table to cat/cow is a lovely way to warm the back.

Slow Gentle Stretching

Be slow and gentle with yourself when moving through your practice. Keep in mind Christ's words to us — *Take my yoke upon you and learn from me, for I am gentle and humble in heart, and you will find rest for your souls.* Move from the warm up into gentle stretching and movement of the joints.

Moderate Repetitive Movements

Gradually build the intensity and heat of the body through moderate repetitive movements.

Increase Intensity of Postures

Increase the energy of your movements and heat the core of the body. Move into more demanding postures and flows.

Transition

Gradually take down the intensity again and move into postures for cool down and rest. Complete the practice with a time of relaxation in resting pose. You may need a blanket in case you become chilled as your body cools down.

At Yahweh Yoga, we generally start our practice resting on our backs, gradually building heat through stretching and core strengthening using twisting supine postures. Then we progress to balancing and standing postures, and increase the intensity through several energetic flows. Then we work our way back down to our mats and finally to resting pose.

General Notes

It is important to keep in mind the yoga principle of *pose and counterpose*. Simply, this is keeping your body in balance in all directions. Anything that you do with or toward the left side of your body you also want to do with or toward the right side with the same intensity and duration. Backward bending postures need to be followed by forward bending postures and vice versa.

Slow, controlled and sustained movements will help you build strength and balance better than rapid or jerky motions. Try to move and breathe into a posture with your limbs energized and controlled; don't flop or fall or bounce into and out of postures. Sustaining and holding postures also helps build strength. Never hold beyond what you can bear comfortably but try to push a little closer to your "own sweet edge" each time. Pain is never good but you need to "feel" the stretch.

Be mindful of your posture and body alignment. Pay careful attention to your teacher's instructions about where your hips are to be facing or the angles of your limbs. Also be careful about twisting the knees. Keep your shoulders down and back; you don't want them hunched up around your neck and ears which is a default position for many of us. Keep your spine straight and long.

Balance is an integral part of many of the postures. Be gracious to yourself and check your balance everyday —it always changes for a multitude of reasons. Usually one side or the other will be better balanced. Your balance in general will improve with regular yoga practice but you still need to be careful.

A flow consists of a series or sequence of postures put together for the purpose of energizing the body. We've included the Sun Salutation as an example of a flow. You will see that this flow includes postures that take you from a prone position on your mat up through standing and balancing and back down to your mat. As you become more comfortable with yoga you will be able to put together your own flows or sequences of postures.

With these guidelines you are ready to start working with the postures in the next section. Do pay careful attention to the instructions and note any cautions or warnings. Work your way through the different types of postures carefully and gradually, keeping in mind the progression of movement outlined above.

When you practice yoga always be careful to listen to your body. There is no competition in yoga so resist the temptation to compare yourself to the person beside you or the pictures in the book. Work to reach your own limit not the example of your classmates. You can seriously injure yourself if you try to compete. Trust me. I've done it, when I've tried to lift my leg just as high as my neighbor or reach as far in a twist as my instructor, instead of respecting my own limit. Practice with your eyes closed as much as possible. There should be no real pain in your yoga practice so learn to discern between stretching yourself and pushing too hard. Maintain steady and comfortable movements and most importantly—*don't forget to breathe.*

Finally, prepare your mind and heart for practice. Ask God to meet you and speak to you. Ask his blessing on your time and his blessing on your body as you seek to care for it. With regular practice your body will move better and feel better. You will walk taller and stand straighter. Imagine the freedom you will feel! Hold these pictures from the Bible in your mind:

> Strengthen the feeble hands,
> steady the knees that give way;
> say to those with fearful hearts,
> "Be strong, do not fear;
> your God will come, ...he will come to save you."

Then will the eyes of the blind be opened

and the ears of the deaf unstopped.

Then will the lame leap like a deer,

and the mute tongue shout for joy.

Water will gush forth in the wilderness

and streams in the desert (Isaiah 35:3-6).

But for you who revere my name, the sun of righteousness will rise with healing in its wings. And you will go out and leap like calves released from the stall (Malachi 4:2).

Imagine strong hands and steady knees! Imagine leaping like a young deer or calf! Imagine a heart warmed by the healing sun of righteousness and overflowing with joy instead of being weighed down by a body in pain. It is within your grasp. The Lord bless you as you seek you to honor him with your body.

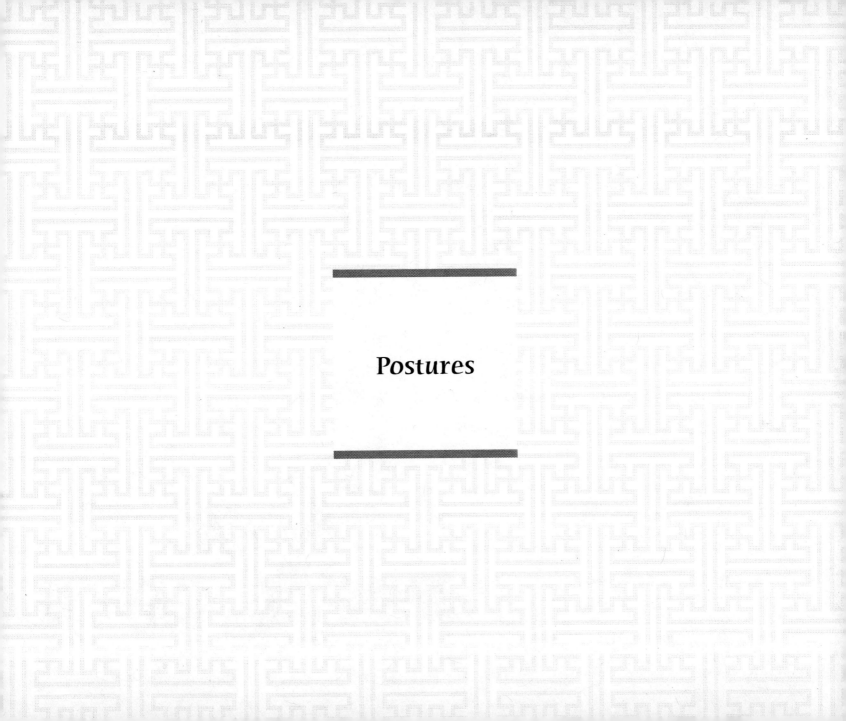

Postures

Boat - WARM UP

Benefits

- Strengthens the abdomen, hip flexors and spine.
- Stimulates the kidneys, thyroid, prostate glands and intestines.
- Helps relieve stress.
- Improves digestion.

Contraindications

- Neck injury; sit with back near a wall to perform pose. While tilting torso back, rest the back of the head on the wall.
- Asthma.
- Diarrhea.
- Headache.
- Heart problems.
- Insomnia.
- Low blood pressure.
- Menstruation.
- Pregnancy.

Common Misalignments

- Shoulders rounding forward.
- Behind sits bone.
- Head forward.
- Lack of muscular and organic energy.

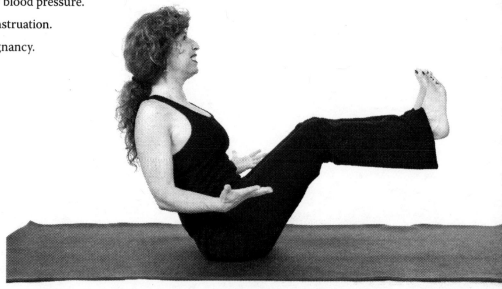

STEP BY STEP

1. Sit on the mat with legs out straight.

2. Press hands on the mat a little behind the hips, shoulders back and wrap around the spine, fingers pointing towards the feet and arms strengthen.

3. Lift up through the top of the sternum and lean back slightly.

4. Bend knees to a 45 degree angle lifting feet off of the floor; feet are active.

5. Come onto sits bone.

6. Stretch arms out along side the legs parallel each other and the floor, palms in and stretch through the fingers.

7. Extend legs out straight, pointing toes and if possible rise above eye level.

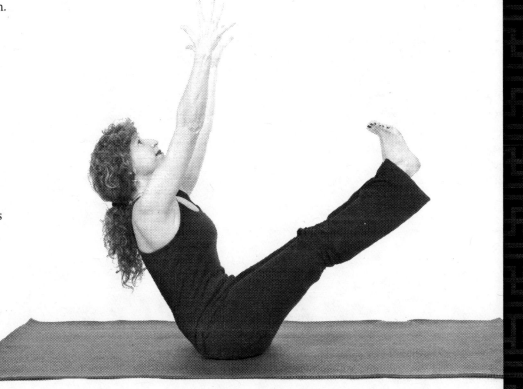

Bridge - WARM UP

STEP BY STEP

1. Lie flat on back; bend knees and set feet parallel on mat as close to sitting bones as possible, hips width apart.

2. Arms placed by the side palms facing down.

3. Inhale and, pressing your inner feet and arms actively into the floor and lift hips.

4. Lift buttocks until the thighs are about parallel to the floor. Knees should be directly over the heels.

5. Lift chin slightly away from sternum and shoulders wrap around the spine as they press into the mat as the sides go long.

Benefits

- Stretches the chest, neck and spine.
- Calms the brain and helps alleviate stress and mild depression.
- Stimulates abdominal organs, lungs and thyroid.
- Rejuvenates tired legs.
- Improves digestion.
- Helps relieve the symptoms of menopause.
- Relieves menstrual discomfort when done supported.
- Reduces anxiety, fatigue, backache, headache and insomnia.
- Therapeutic for asthma, high blood pressure, osteoporosis and sinusitis.

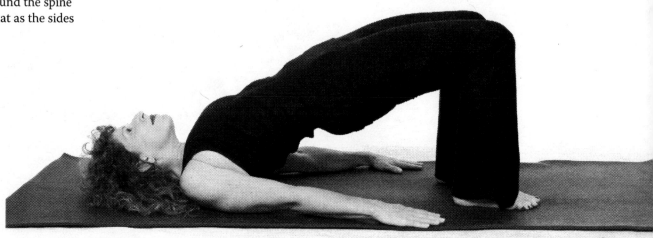

Contraindications

- Neck injury. Avoid this pose unless you are practicing under the supervision of an experienced teacher.

Common Misalignments

- Chin tucked flattening the neck.
- Pulling shoulders away from ears.
- Feet and knees misaligned.
- Clenching of glut muscles.

Modifications

- Use block under sacrum for support.
- Use block between thighs to draw thighs together.

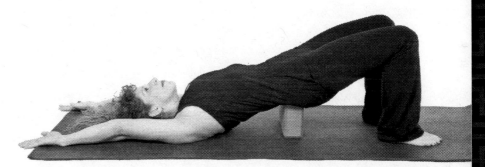

block under sacrum

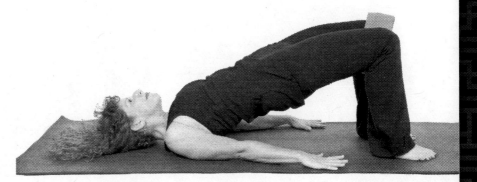

block between thighs

Butterfly - WARM UP

STEP BY STEP

1. Sit with legs out straight. Inhale.

2. Exhale, bend knees, pull heels toward the pelvis, drop knees out to the sides and press the soles of the feet together as if the bottoms of the feet are kissing.

3. Bring heels as close to pelvis as comfortably as possible.

4. Sit up straight; pubis in front and the tailbone in the back are equidistant from the floor.

5. Firm the sacrum and shoulder blades against the back and lengthen the front torso through the top of the sternum.

Benefits

- Stretches the inner thigh and groins.
- Strengthens abdominal muscles.
- Stimulates abdominal organs, ovaries and prostate gland, bladder and kidneys.
- Stimulates the heart and improves general circulation.
- Helps relieve mild depression, anxiety and fatigue.
- Soothes menstrual discomfort and sciatica.
- Helps relieve the symptoms of menopause.
- Therapeutic for flat feet, high blood pressure, infertility and asthma.

Contraindications

- Groin or knee injury: Only perform this pose with support under outer thighs.

Common Misalignments

- Pelvis foundation.
- Lumbar kyphosis.
- Pushing knees down.
- Sickled feet.
- Shoulders and head forward.

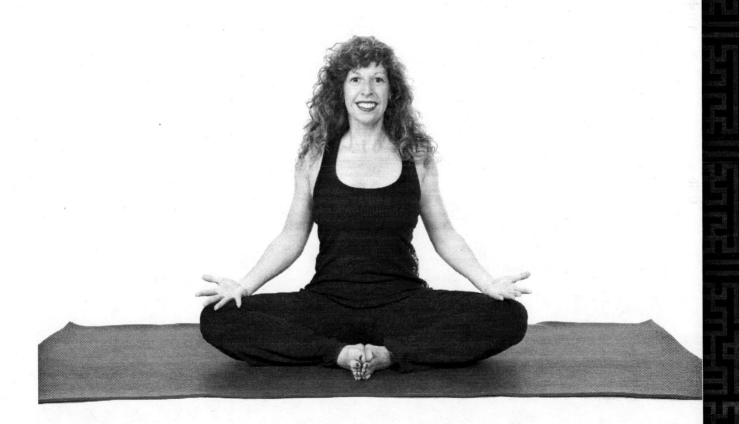

CHRISTIAN YOGA ✣ *Postures*

Cat / Cow - WARM UP

STEP BY STEP

1. Come into Table Pose.

2. Knees under hips and wrist under shoulders.

3. Allow the breath to guide the movement of the body into the poses.

4. Inhale as the belly drops, heart and head lift and the tailbone presses up and out. (Cow Pose)

5. Head draws down and chin tucks. (Cat Pose)

6. Exhale as back arches and belly button draws towards the spine.

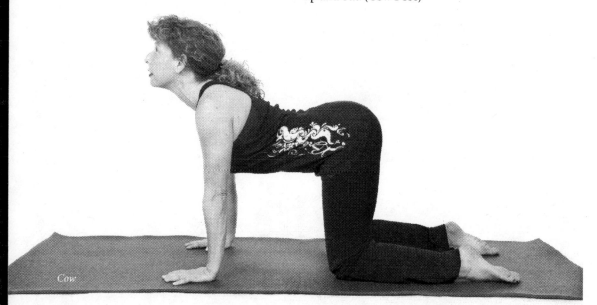

Cow

Benefits

- Strengthens abs and back.
- Good way to connect to correct breathing.

Contraindications

- Carpal tunnel syndrome.
- Neck injuries.

Common Misalignments

- Hands turned in and/or knuckles not connected.
- Elbows bent.
- Upper arms rolled in.
- Legs and/or toes asleep.

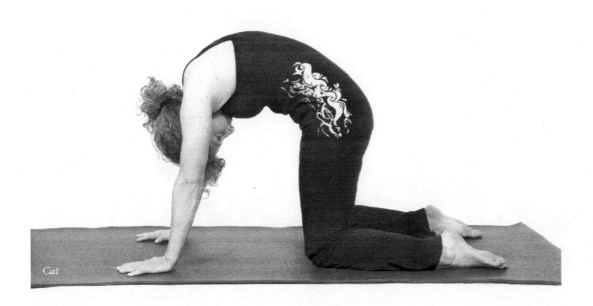

Cat

Fish - WARM UP

STEP BY STEP

1. Start by lying down on the back.

2. Tuck forearms and elbows up close to the sides of the torso.

3. Palms slightly under the seat. Elbows and forearms are pressed down on the mat. Then press scapulas into the back and with an inhale, lift upper torso and head away from the floor.

4. Head releases back to the floor as heart rises.

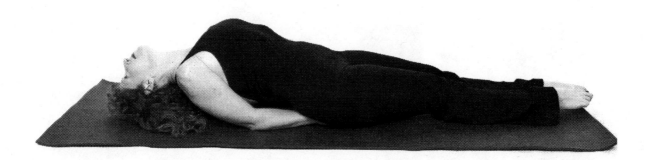

Benefits

- Stretches the deep hip flexor and the muscles between the ribs.
- Stretches and stimulates the muscles of the belly, throat and the front of the neck.
- Strengthens the muscles of the upper back and back of neck.
- Improves posture.
- Helps relieve asthma.
- Aids to digestion

Contraindications

- High of low blood pressure.
- Migraine.
- Insomnia.
- Serious lower back pain or neck injury.

Common Misalignments

- Neck bent instead of a long gentle curve.
- Legs inactive.
- Legs outer spiraled.
- Lack of should and/or pelvic loop.

Forward Bend - WARM UP

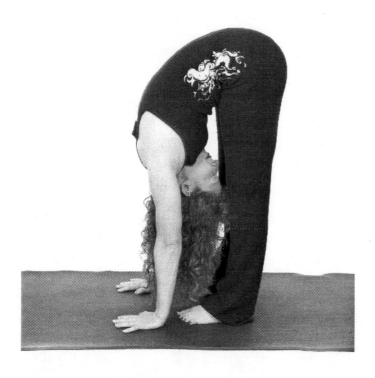

STEP BY STEP

1. Stand in Mountain with hands on hips.

2. Exhale and bend forward from the hip joints, not from waist.

3. Descend drawing the front of the torso out of the groins and open the space between the pubis and top sternum.

4. Move fully into the position while lengthening the front torso.

5. The knees should be straight and the palms or finger tips on the floor slightly in front or beside the feet. You may use a block or press your hands into your thighs if you can not reach the floor.

6. Press heels firmly into the floor and lift the sitting bones towards the ceiling.

7. Shins In Thighs Out.

8. Allow the head to hang from the root of the neck, which is deep in the upper back, between the shoulder blades.

Benefits

- Calms the brain and helps relieve stress and mild depression.
- Stimulates the liver and kidneys.
- Stretches the hamstrings, calves and hips.
- Strengthens the thighs and knees.
- Improves digestion.
- Helps relieve the symptoms of menopause.
- Reduces fatigue and anxiety.
- Relieves Headache and insomnia.
- Therapeutic for asthma, high blood pressure, infertility, osteoporosis and sinusitis.

Contraindications

- Unmedicated high blood pressure.
- Detached retina, weak eye capillaries, glaucoma, conjunctivitis or any inflammation of the eyes or ears.
- Recent or chronic injury or inflammation of back, shoulders or knees.

Common Misalignments

- Too much of a curve in the back.
- Setting the gaze towards the earth.
- Acute sciatica (with inflammation).

Modification

- Interlace fingers behind back, lift arms, pulling elbows towards each other behind back.

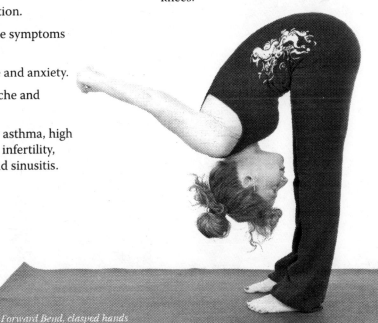

Forward Bend, clasped hands

Mountain - WARM UP

STEP BY STEP

1. Stand with feet hips distance apart, second toes should be parallel and four corners of the feet pressed into the earth.

2. Lift and spread the toes and release one at a time.

3. Gently rock side to side and back and forth until weight is balanced evenly on both feet. Legs should be firmly rooted into the earth.

4. Tornado the legs feeling a spiraling effect from the base of the feet upward to the top of the crown... Shins in Thighs Out... thighs tighten as knee caps lift up the thigh.

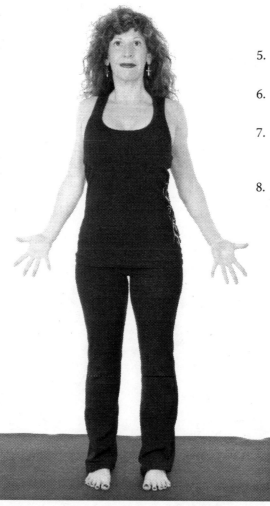

5. Tuck tailbone and lift pubis toward the naval.

6. Sides go long and allow spine to rise up.

7. Shoulder blades press into back and then release down back. Heart lifts. Arms down by side.

8. Body parts stack one on top of the other ending with the head in line with the middle of pelvis.

Benefits

- Improves posture
- Strengthens thighs, knees, and ankles
- Firms abdomen and buttocks
- Relieves sciatica
- Reduces flat feet
- Foundation pose for all standing poses

Contraindications

- Headache
- Insomnia
- Low blood pressure

Common Misalignments

- Foundation: Feet not parallel, too wide/narrow of stance, weight not balanced in feet.
- Lack of muscular energy, muscles not grabbed onto bones.
- Thighs, shoulders or head forward.
- Palms facing back.

Seated Forward Bend - WARM UP

STEP BY STEP

1. Set foundation, sit up straight with legs out long, shoulders back and heart lifts, feet flex.

2. Strengthen thigh muscles.

3. Inner spiral, widen thighs and anchor inner edge of legs to floor.

4. Extend from pelvis core out through feet and up through crown of head.

5. Then hinge at hips forward and draw your heart down toward the thighs.

6. Lengthen through the top of the crown.

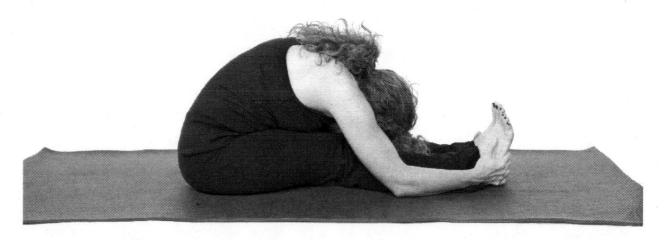

Benefits

- Foundational pose for all seated postures.
- Strengthens and improves endurance of back, leg and arm muscles.
- Opens chest, hips and groin.
- Tones abdominal muscles.
- Increases circulation.
- Great for spine.

Contraindications

- Unmedicated high blood pressure.
- Recent or chronic injury or inflammation of back, shoulders or knees.
- Acute sciatica (with inflammation).

Common Misalignments

- Lumbar kyphosis.
- Curving the back.
- Head tucked in too much.
- Shoulders forward.
- Leg muscles relaxed.

Stacked Logs - WARM UP

STEP BY STEP

1. Come to a seated pose, shoulders back and sides long.
2. Lifting through your crown gain length in the spine.
3. Stack heals and knees.
4. Activate feet and hands to the heart.

Benefits

- Opens hips and stretches the outer hip muscles.
- Strengthens feet and ankles.

Contraindications

- Knee injury.

Common Misalignments

- Feet sickled or asleep.
- Lower back kyphosis.

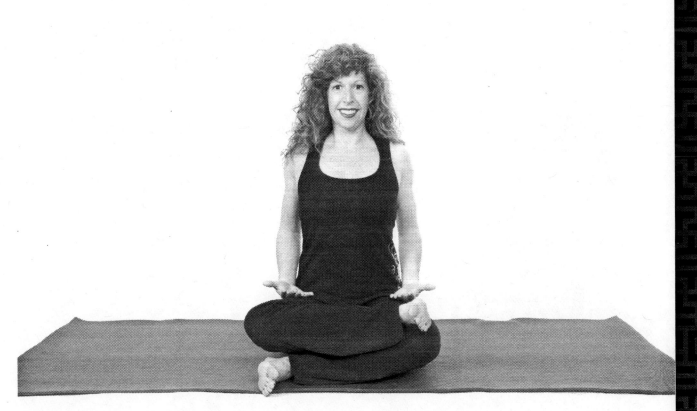

Staff - WARM UP

STEP BY STEP

1. Set foundation, sit up straight with legs out long, shoulders back and heart lifts, feet flex. Spread toes.

2. Strengthen thigh muscles.

3. Inner spiral, widen thighs and anchor inner edge of legs to floor.

4. Extend from pelvis core out through feet and up through crown of head.

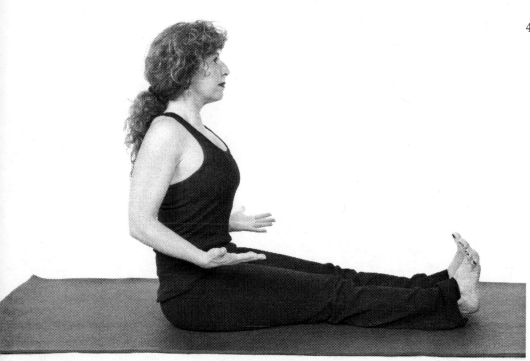

Benefits

- Foundational pose from all seated postures.
- Strengthens and improves endurance of back, leg and arm muscles.
- Opens chest, hips and groin.
- Tones abdominal muscles.
- Increases circulation.

Contraindications

- If the body is leaning back it may be because tight hamstrings are dragging the sitting bones toward the knees and the back of the pelvis toward the floor. If that is happening elevate pelvis by sitting on a blanket.

Common Misalignments

- Torso leaning back.
- Shoulders forward.
- Leg muscles relaxed.

Table - WARM UP

STEP BY STEP

1. Come onto hands and knees.
2. Hands are placed under the shoulders and are active.
3. Knees are under the hips and legs are active.
4. Core is tightened and gaze is to the mat.

Benefits

- Strengthens abs and back.
- Helps teach good hand foundation.

Contraindications

- Carpal tunnel syndrome.

Common Misalignments

- Hands turned in and/or knuckles not connected.
- Elbows bent.
- Upper arms rolled in.
- Shins out or asleep.

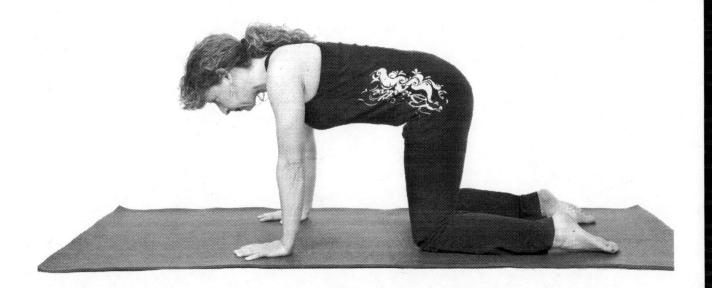

CHRISTIAN YOGA ✢ Postures

Bottom of a Push Up - FLOW

STEP BY STEP

1. From Plank Pose tighten and lift thighs and waist, shoulder blades on the back.

2. Slightly jet forward and lower down until arms are at a 90 degree angle and body hovering a few inches above the mat.

3. Elbows hug into the sides of the body, shoulders stay broad and gaze is towards the mat.

Benefits

- Strengthens the arms and wrists.
- Tones the abdomen and builds core strength.
- Energizes the body.

Contraindications

- Carpal Tunnel Syndrome.
- Pregnancy.

Common Misalignments

- Hands misaligned.
- Elbows out.
- Forearm not perpendicular to the floor.
- Shoulder heads dipped forward.
- Abdomen drooped.

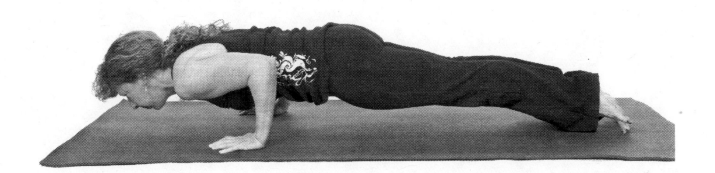

Cobra - FLOW

STEP BY STEP

1. Lay on belly, spread hands and place under the shoulders, back by rib cage. Hug elbows back into body. Downward Dog hands claw at mat.

2. Spread toes and firmly press tops of feet, thighs and pubis into the mat.

3. Inhale, head and chest lift as sides lengthen. Pressing mat away begin to straighten arms. Lift as high as possible keeping hips and leg connected to mat.

4. Tailbone presses towards the pubis and the pubis presses towards the naval. Firm but don't harden buttocks.

5. Wrap shoulders around the spin and lift up through the heart. Head up and gaze forward.

Benefits

- Strengthens the spine.
- Stretches the chest, lungs, shoulders and abdomen.
- Firms the buttocks.
- Stimulates abdominal organs.
- Helps relieve stress and fatigue.
- Opens the heart and lungs.
- Soothes sciatica.
- Therapeutic for asthma

Contraindications

- Back injury.
- Carpal Tunnel Syndrome.
- Headache.
- Pregnancy.

Common Misalignments

- Palms in and elbows out.
- Hands and/or feet asleep.
- Feet sickled.
- Shoulders forward.
- Hard traps.

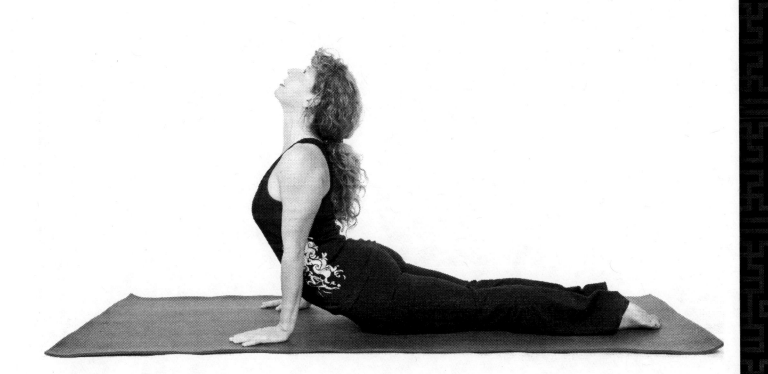

CHRISTIAN YOGA ✠ *Postures*

Crow - FLOW

STEP BY STEP

1. Come into a squat, hands on the mat under shoulders; wrist parallel and fingers clawing on mat.

2. Knees to the back of the upper arms as close to the arm pit as possible.

3. Gaze forward ahead of fingers, rock forward getting the weight into the fingers.

4. Lift one foot at a time while flexing foot and spreading toes. Tailbone lifts.

5. Hug forearms, feet, legs and knees to the middle and then straighten arms.

Benefits

- Strengthens arms and wrists.
- Stretches the upper back.
- Strengthens the abdominal muscles.
- Opens groins.
- Tones the abdominal organs.

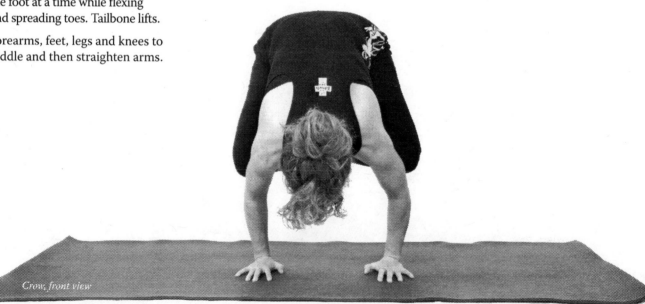

Crow, front view

Contraindications

- Carpal tunnel syndrome.
- Pregnancy.

Common Misalignments

- Hands misaligned.
- Lack of hugging to the middle with hands, forearms and legs.
- Gaze towards the feet.
- Feet asleep.

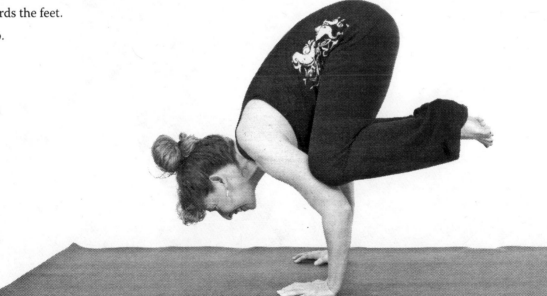

Crow, side view

Dolphin - FLOW

STEP BY STEP

1. From Downward-Facing Dog come onto forearms.

2. Elbows come under the shoulders and forearms extend straight out. Wrists are shoulders width apart and palms on the mat.

3. Heart melts as gravity takes your heart and body down.

4. Gaze is between the hands as legs walk in towards the body.

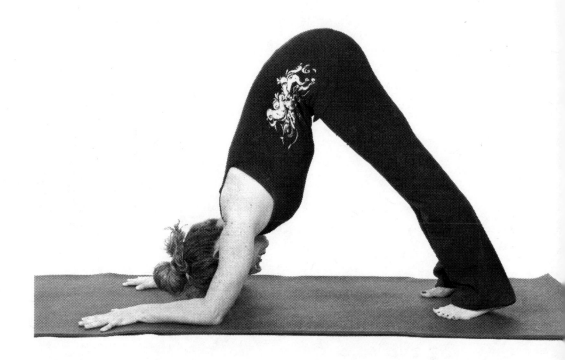

Benefits

- Strengthens the shoulders, arms and back.
- Stretches the shoulders, neck, chest and belly.
- Improves sense of balance.
- Calms the brain and helps relieve stress and mild depression.

Contraindications

- Back, shoulder or neck injuries.
- Headache.
- Heart condition.
- High blood pressure.
- Menstruation.

Common Misalignments

- Elbows are wide.
- Wrist width is narrow.
- Pushing away from the earth, losing shoulder loop.
- Lack of muscular energy in legs.
- Lack of kidney loop.

Downward-Facing Dog - FLOW

STEP BY STEP

1. Come onto the floor on your hands and knees.

2. Set up proper alignment; knees under hips, hands under shoulders and slightly wider than shoulders width, wrist creases parallel, fingers spread and claw into mat.

3. Inhale and squeeze arms together, firm shoulder blades against back, tuck toes and allow hips to rise. Pressing the earth away from you.

4. Heals stretch to or onto the floor.

5. Head stays between the arms not dangling free.

6. The heart is reaching for the thighs.

Benefits

• Calms the brain and helps relieve stress and mild depression.

• Energizes the body.

• Stretches the shoulders, hamstrings, calves, arches and hands.

• Strengthens the arms and legs.

• Helps relieve symptoms of menopause.

• Helps prevent osteoporosis.

• Improves digestion.

• Relieves headache, insomnia, back pain and fatigue.

• Therapeutic for high blood pressure, asthma, flat feet, sciatica, sinusitis.

Contraindications

• Carpal Tunnel Syndrome.

• Diarrhea.

• *Pregnancy*: Do not do this pose late-term.

• High blood pressure or headache: Support your head on a bolster or block, ears level between arms.

Common Misalignments

- Foundation: Hands turned in, fingertips up, metacarpals lifted.
- Foundation: Feet too wide, turned in, rolled out.
- Foundation: Too short of a stance.
- Straight knees but round back.
- Inner spiral upper arms, resulting in bent elbows, shoulders at ears, and scapula off back.

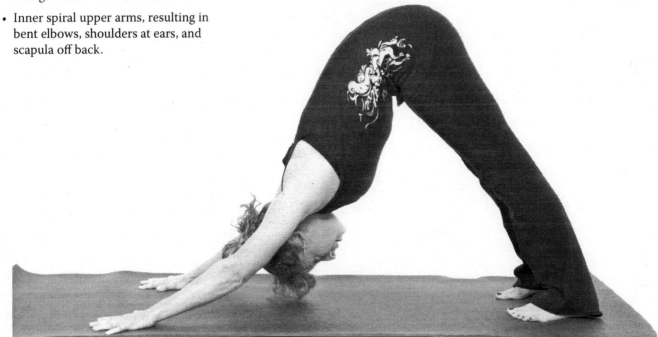

Half Moon - FLOW

STEP BY STEP

1. Start in Standing Forward Bend (Triangle, Warrior 2/3 or Side Angle) and extend one leg up parallel to the mat.

2. Hand places on the mat 6-8 inches in front of the same side foot.

3. Hips stack one on top of the other as other arm extends up.

4. Fingers spread and foot flexes.

5. Tuck tailbone under and tighten core.

6. Gaze is down at the hand on the mat, straight forward or up at the extended arm.

Benefits

- Strengthens the abdomen, ankles, thighs, buttocks and spine.

- Stretches the groins, hamstrings, calves, shoulders, chest and spine.

- Improves coordination and sense of balance.

- Helps relieve stress and improves digestion.

Contraindications

- Someone with neck problems should not look up towards the extended hand; continue looking straight ahead and keep both sides of the neck evenly long.

- Headache or migraine.

- Low blood pressure.

- Diarrhea.

- Insomnia.

Common Misalignments

- Foot turned, not on four corners, knee not tracking in the direction of the toe.

- Lack of muscular energy.

- Not enough outer spiral in standing leg.

- Lack of shoulder loop.

- Imbalance of muscular and organic energy.

- Coming out carelessly.

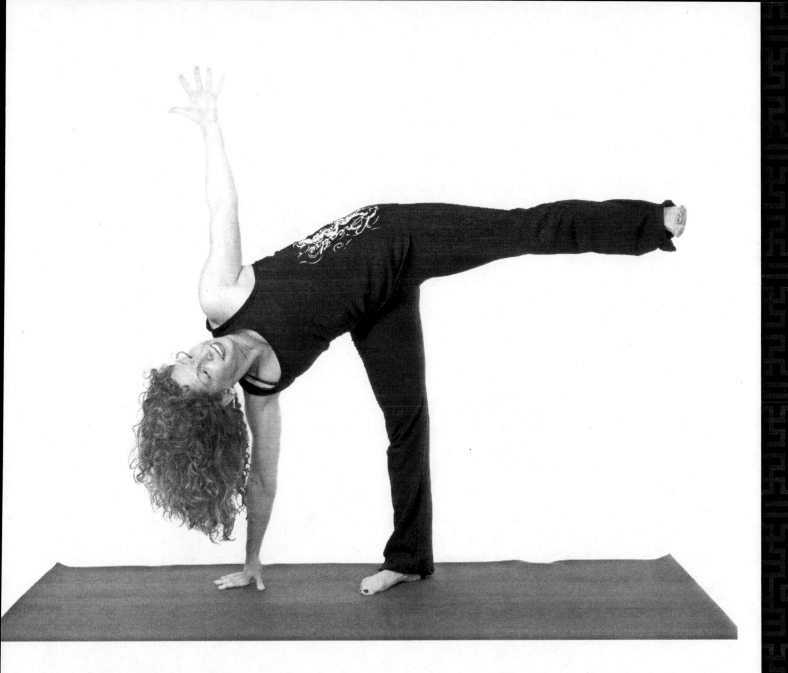

Lunge - FLOW

STEP BY STEP

1. From Mountain Pose step one foot back (basic).

2. From Downward Dog take foot to hand (advanced).

3. Hands on outside of feet, come onto fingers, elbows bent and shoulders back.

4. Front knee comes over ankle by wiggling back foot back.

5. Lift back inner thigh up and hug legs in together.

6. Inhale back into body and exhale and soften behind heart.

7. Head up and looking forward.

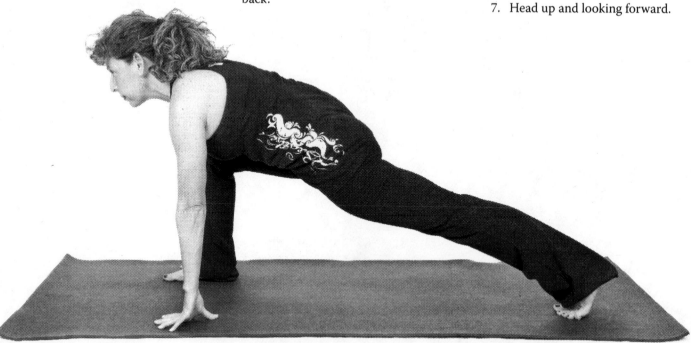

Benefits

- Stimulates digestion.
- Stretches the shoulders, chest, and groins.
- Strengthens arches, knees, thighs, calves and ankles.
- Increases muscular endurance.
- Relieves symptoms of sciatica.

Contraindications

- Knee injuries, know knee alignment.

Common Misalignments

- Front knee going past ankle.
- Foundation, too short of stance and lounge not deep.
- Back knee dropped.
- Hands turned in, flat hands and round upper back.
- Head hung down.

Open to HIS Grace - FLOW

STEP BY STEP

1. Stand with feet hips distance apart, second toes should be parallel and four corners of the feet pressed into the earth.

2. Lift and spread the toes and release one at a time.

3. Gently rock side to side and back and forth until weight is balanced evenly on both feet. Legs should be firmly rooted into the earth.

4. Tornado the legs... Shins in Thighs Out... thighs tighten as knee caps lift up the thigh.

5. Tuck tailbone and lift pubis toward the naval.

6. Sides go long and allow spine to rise up.

7. Lift your arms over the head and your heart lifts. Left your heart as an offering to our Lord. Creating a slight backbend.

8. Open your arms a bit wider than your shoulders.

9. Fingers spread.

10. Drop head back just slightly. Make sure you can still swallow or your head is back too far.

Benefits

- Improves posture
- Strengthens thighs, knees, and ankles
- Firms abdomen and buttocks
- Relieves sciatica
- Good for your shoulders and lower back

Contraindications

- Headache
- Insomnia
- Low blood pressure

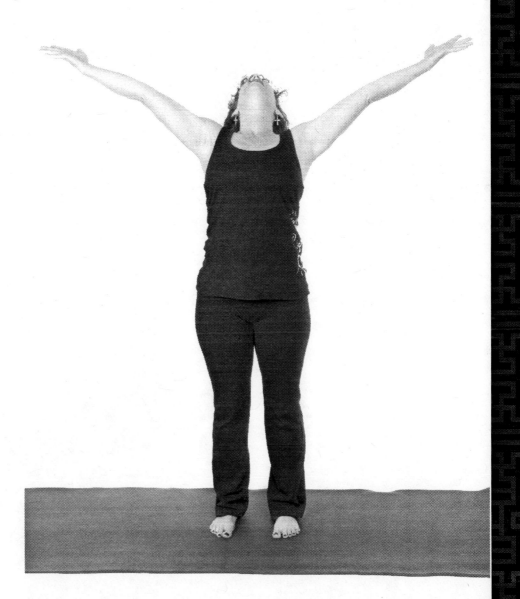

Common Misalignments

- Foundation: Feet not parallel, too wide/narrow of stance, weight not balanced in feet.

- Lack of muscular energy, muscles not grabbed onto bones.

- Thighs, shoulders or head forward.

- Head dropped back too far.

Plank - FLOW

STEP BY STEP

1. From a Forward Bend press hands into the earth and walk or jump feet back.

2. Fingers spread and claw at mat. The wrists are in line with each other and under the shoulder.

3. Core tightens as muscles wrap around the bones and tailbone tucks.

4. Actively pull your belly button toward the spine.

5. Waist lifts as heart melts.

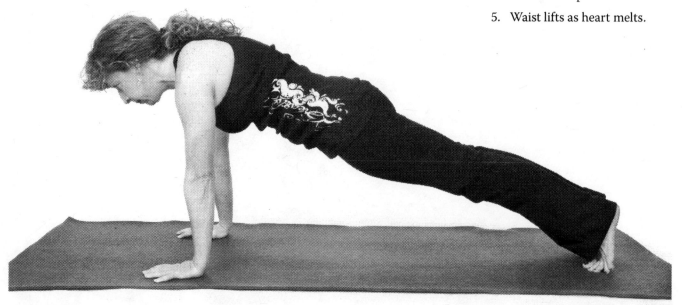

Benefits

• Strengthens arms, wrists and spine.

• Tones abdomen.

Contraindications

• Carpal Tunnel Syndrome.

Common Misalignments

• Hands misaligned.

• Too short of a stance so back rounds or hips lift.

• Forearms not perpendicular to floor.

• Shoulder heads dipped forward, scapula not on back.

• Abdomen droops.

Pyramid - FLOW

STEP BY STEP

1. From Mountain Pose (Lunge, Triangle or Downward-Facing Dog) draw leg back, heel to the mat and back toes are facing forward.

2. Front knees are in line with toes.

3. Hips and shoulders point forward and fold at the hips drawing the head to the knee.

4. Activate both legs equally by pulling knee caps up and hips forward.

5. Hands on the mat.

Benefits

- Opens the chest.
- Calms the brain.
- Stretches the spine, shoulders, hips and hamstrings.
- Strengthens the legs, feet and ankles.
- Stimulates the abdominal organs and thyroid.
- Improves posture and sense of balance.
- Improves digestion.

Contraindications

- Back injuries; don't fold all the way down. Use a wall if desired.
- Pregnancy.

Common Misalignments

- Feet turned, not for corners.
- Feet in line, back foot too turned out.
- Hyper extending or bending knees.
- Lack of muscular energy.
- Hips and shoulders not to the front.

Side Angle Stretch - FLOW

STEP BY STEP

1. From Warrior 2 with right leg forward, place right hand by the right foot.

2. Then tuck tail bone under and roll your shoulders back.

3. Extend the left arm up over the head.

4. Take gaze up to the left hand.

5. Spread the fingers and lift the heart.

Benefits

• Stimulates digestion.

• Stretches the shoulders, chest, and groins.

• Strengthens arches, knees, thighs, calves and ankles.

• Increases muscular endurance.

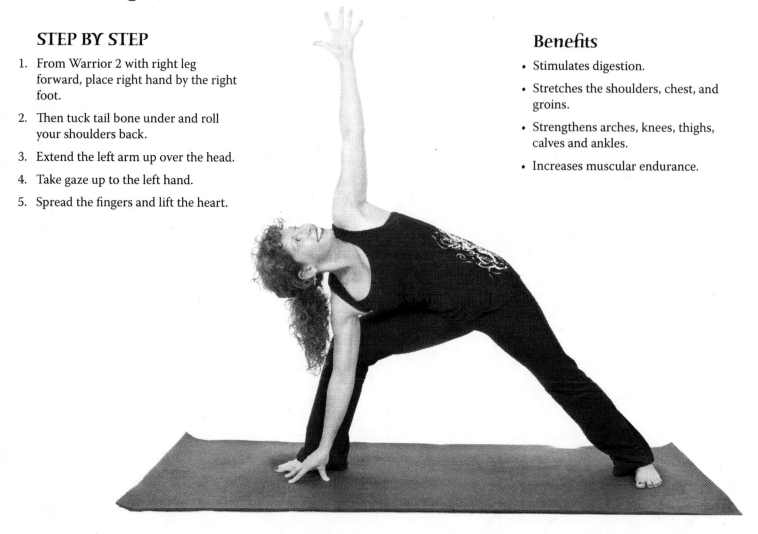

Contraindications

• Knee injury

Common Misalignments

• Leaning forward

• Leaning too much into front knee

• Tail bone out

• Gaze is down

Modifications

• Take the bind by inserting bottom arm from the front of the body under thigh and reaching behind back by bending the elbow. The top arm reaches behind the back to grip the bottom hand.

• If your hands do not meet yet, use a strap or towel to make the connection with the hands.

• Extend the top arm over the head.

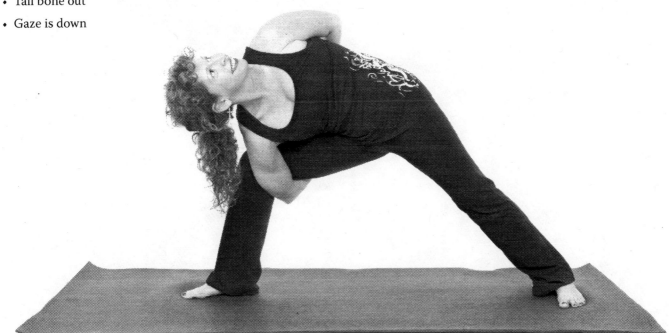

Side Arm Balance - FLOW

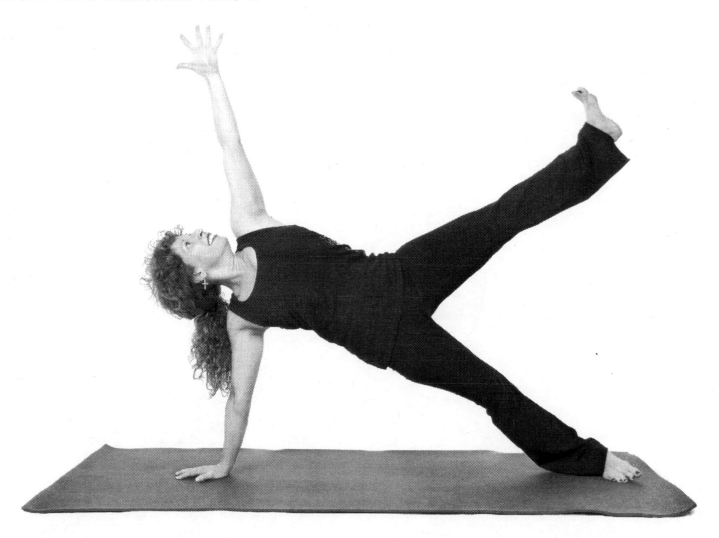

STEP BY STEP

1. Come into Plank Pose and place one hand under the face so that hand is in front of the shoulder.

2. Feet become active, toes spread and press into the inner edges of the feet as hips draw up off the mat and other hands rests on the hip or extends straight up.

3. Heart opens as thighs strengthen while extending through inside of leg and inner foot presses towards the floor.

4. Gaze is up at extended hand.

5. You may also do this pose with one knee on the mat. Use the same knee down as what hand is on the mat.

6. Advanced you may want to lift the top leg up.

Benefits

• Strengthens the arms, belly and legs.

• Stretches and strengthens the wrists.

• Stretches the backs of the legs (in full version of the pose).

• Improves sense of balance.

Contraindications

• Students with serious wrist, elbow or shoulder injuries should avoid this pose.

Common Misalignments

• Hand misaligned; under or behind shoulder.

• Feet and/or leg muscles asleep.

• Lack of shoulder loop.

• Head forward.

Sphinx - FLOW

STEP BY STEP

1. Lay on belly, elbows under the shoulder, wrists coming straight out from elbows with forearms resting on the earth and hands down.

2. Elbows and fingers are inline with each other.

3. Spread fingers, knuckles and finger tips press down on mat.

4. Thighs become active, spread toes and press feet into floor.

5. Shoulders back and hearts lifts off the mat.

Benefits

- Strengthens back, arms, shoulders, legs and wrists.
- Stretches chest, lungs, shoulders and abdomen.
- Firms the buttocks.
- Improves posture.
- Stimulates digestion and circulation.
- Helps relieve stress and fatigue.
- Opens the heart, throat and increases lung capacity.
- Soothes sciatica.
- Therapeutic for asthma.

Contraindications

- Back injury.
- Carpal Tunnel Syndrome.
- Headache.
- Pregnancy.
-

Common Misalignments

- Wrists and elbows in.
- Hands and/or legs asleep.
- Feet sickled.
- Shoulders forward.

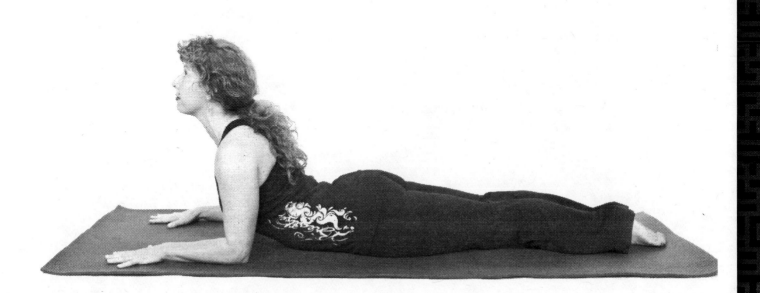

CHRISTIAN YOGA ✠ Postures

Triangle - FLOW

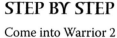

STEP BY STEP

1. Come into Warrior 2 Pose and then straighten the front leg.

2. Extend the torso over the front leg, bending at the hip joint not the waist. Rest extended hand on the shin or the mat behind or in front of the calf.

3. Press into the back foot lengthening all the way up through the side and opening up through the heart. Tailbone tucks.

4. Extend the back arm up towards the ceiling, fingers active. Keep arm in line with the shoulders.

5. Keep head in a neutral position or gently gaze upwards towards hand.

Benefits

• Stretches and strengthens the thighs, knees and ankles.

• Stretches the hips, groins, hamstrings, calves, shoulders, chest and spine.

• Stimulates the abdominal organs.

• Helps relieve stress.

• Improves digestion.

• Helps relieve the symptoms of menopause.

• Relieves backache especially through second trimester of pregnancy.

• Therapeutic for anxiety, flat feet, infertility, neck pain, osteoporosis and sciatica.

Contraindications

- Diarrhea.
- Headache.
- Low blood pressure.
- Heart condition; practice on the wall and keep top arm on the hip.
- High blood pressure; turn the gaze downward in the final pose.
- Neck problems; don't turn the head to look upward, continue looking straight ahead and keep both sides of the neck evenly long.

Common Misalignments

- Feet turned, not four corners.
- Feet not in line, back foot is too turned out.
- Lack of muscular energy.
- Knees bent or hyper extended.
- Hips in same plane as feet causing front knee to cave to midline.

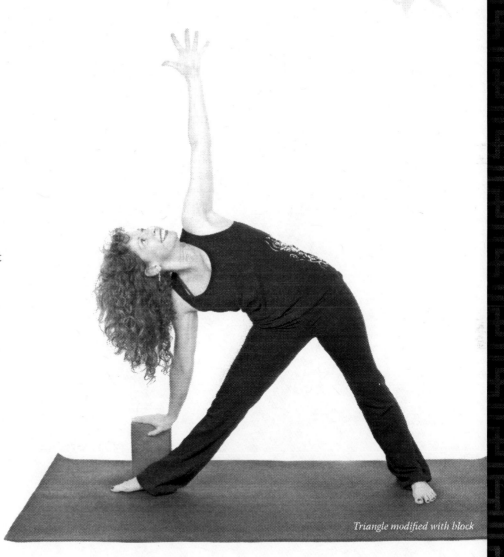

Triangle modified with block

Warrior One - FLOW

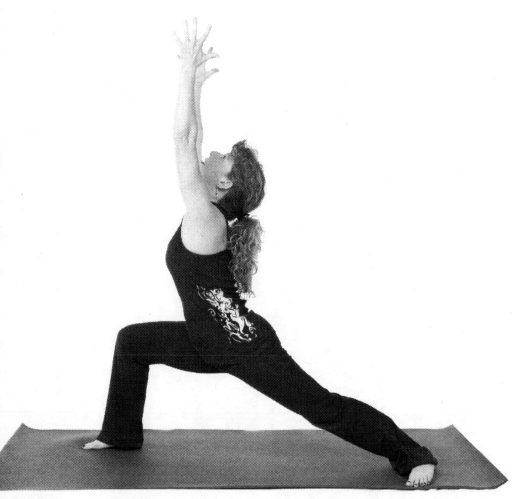

STEP BY STEP

1. From Mountain Pose (Lunge or Downward Dog) step straight back and turn back toes out slightly.

2. Back leg is active as heel presses into the floor, thigh draws up. Bend the front knee over the heel and in line with toes. Shin should be perpendicular to the floor. Try to bring right thigh parallel to the floor.

3. Hips and shoulders square off to the front of the room.

4. Fingers are active and spread as arms lift up. Shoulder bones are pressed back into the sockets and heart rises and arms lift over the head and come back by the ears. Palms turn in to face each other; pinkies turn in slightly if desired to activate triceps.

5. Gaze is forward or tilted back to look at the fingers.

Benefits

- Stretches the chest, lungs, shoulders, neck, belly and groin.
- Strengthens the shoulders, arms and back muscles.
- Stretches and strengthens the thighs, calves, arches and ankles.
- Increases muscular endurance.

Contraindications

- High blood pressure.
- Heart problems.
- Students with shoulder problems should keep their raised arms parallel or slightly wider than parallel to each other.
- Students with neck problems should keep their head in a neutral position and not look up at the hands.

Common Misalignments

- Feet turned out, not on four corners.
- Feet in line and /or back foot too turned out.
- Back knee is bent.
- Most of the weight is in the front leg.
- Hips and shoulders are not squared to the front.
- Lack of shoulder loop.

Warrior Two - FLOW

STEP BY STEP

1. From a Standing Wide Leg Straddle raise arms parallel to the mat, actively reaching out to each side and palms down.

2. Turn back foot out 90 degrees lining up the heel of the front foot with the arch of the back foot.

3. Bend into the front knee bringing it line with the toes and over the heel.

4. Lengthen and tighten through the back leg, tail bone tucks under and sink into the pose. Back leg and front leg should be equally active.

5. Lengthen through the top of the head, draw shoulders back, arms slightly relaxed and gaze through the front middle finger

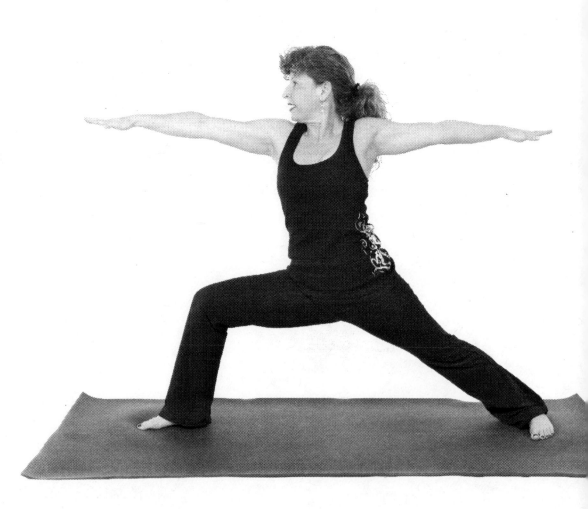

196

Benefits

- Strengthens and stretches the legs, arches of feet and ankles.
- Stretches the groins, chest, lungs and shoulders.
- Stimulates abdominal organ and circulation.
- Increases stamina and lung capacity.
- Increases muscular endurance.
- Relieves backaches, especially through second trimester of pregnancy.
- Therapeutic for carpal tunnel syndrome, flat feet, infertility, osteoporosis and sciatica.

Contraindications

- Diarrhea.
- High blood pressure.
- Neck problems; don't turn head to look over the front hand, continue to look straight ahead with both sides of the neck lengthened evenly.

Common Misalignments

- Feet turned, not on four corners.
- Feet not in line, back foot turned out too much.
- Back knee is bent.
- Most of the weight is in the front leg and/or body is leaning forward.
- Hips in the same plane as feet causing the front knee to cave into the midline.
- Lack of shoulder loop.
- Femur bone is forward

Warrior Three - FLOW

STEP BY STEP

1. From Standing Forward Bend balance on one leg and draw other leg straight back and torso parallel to the floor. Toes are faced down.

2. Front foot is firmly planted on the mat; leg is straight and spirals out. Back foot is flexed and leg has inner spiral. Hips are parallel to the mat. Core is tight.

3. Extend arms out straight in front, palms facing each other and fingers alive. Creating a line from the tips of the fingers through the flexed foot that is parallel to the mat. (Arms can also be interlaced reaching behind you, at waist, or in airplane with palms facing down)

Benefits

- Strengthens the feet, ankles, legs, shoulders and back muscles.
- Tones the abdomen.
- Increases muscular endurance, circulation, stamina and lung capacity.
- Stretches the hips and groin.
- Improves balance and posture.

Contraindications

- Foot turned and/or not on four corners.
- Lack of muscular energy and/or knees bent.
- Hips not parallel to the mat.
- Lack of shoulder loop.
- Torso and back leg not parallel to the mat.

Common Misalignments

- Heart leading down and body leaning forward.
- Not properly setting down foot foundation and loosing balance

Modifications

- Arms can also be interlaced reaching behind you, at waist, or in airplane with palms facing down.

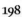

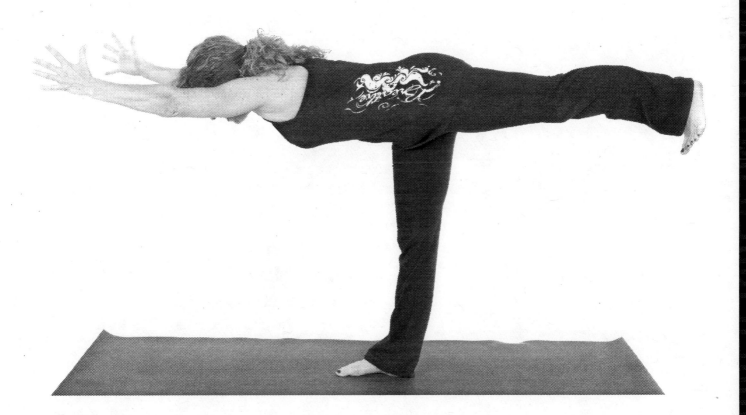

Wild Thing - FLOW

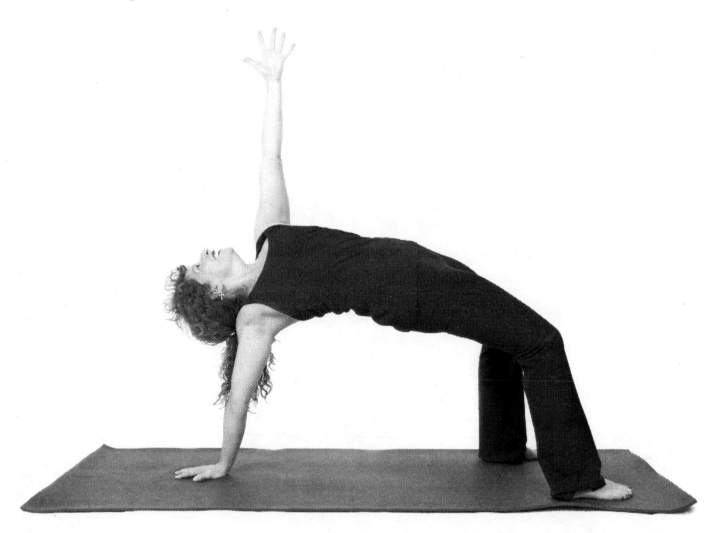

STEP BY STEP

1. Come into Plank Pose and place one hand under the face so that hand is in front of the shoulder.

2. Turn the body to stack hips on top of each other.

3. Feet become active, toes spread and press into the inner edges of the feet as hips draw up and other hands rests on the hip or extends straight up.

4. Heart opens as thighs strengthen while extending through inside of leg and inner foot presses towards the floor.

5. Gaze is up.

6. Lift top leg straight up. Flex the foot.

7. Then drop the leg behind you, curving the back and rolling the shoulder back to lift the heart.

8. Turn the body back over into Plank Pose to finish the series.

Benefits

- Strengthens the back, arms, belly and legs.

- Stretches and strengthens the wrists.

- Improves sense of balance.

Contraindications

- Students with serious wrist, elbow or shoulder injuries should avoid this pose.

Common Misalignments

- Hand misaligned; behind shoulder.

- Feet and/or leg muscles asleep.

- Lack of shoulder loop.

- Head forward.

Bow - COOL DOWN

STEP BY STEP

1. Lie on belly, chin to mat and arms down by the side with palms facing up.

2. Bend at the knees bringing heels as close to the buttocks as possible, wrap shoulders around the spine and reach back with hands taking hold of the ankles or upper feet.

3. Draw knees towards each other and maintain hips width apart for duration of pose.

4. Spread the toes and press feet into the hands.

5. Inhale and strongly lift the heels away from the buttocks and, at the same time, lift the thighs away from the mat. Upper torso and head lift.

6. Knees are magnetized together, upper thighs and heels continue to lift, shoulder blades press against the back and heart opens. Shoulders drop away from the ears and gaze forward.

7. Breathe into the back of the torso.

Benefits

- Stretches the entire front of the body, ankles, things, groin, abdomen, chest, throat and deep hip flexors.

- Strengthens the back muscles.

- Improves posture.

- Stimulates the organs, abdomen and neck.

Contraindications

- Pregnancy.
- Knee injury.
- High or low blood pressure.
- Migraine.
- Insomnia.
- Serious lower back or neck injury.

Common Misalignments

- Knees flaring out.
- Feet asleep.
- Shoulders forward.
- Lack of tailbone scooping.

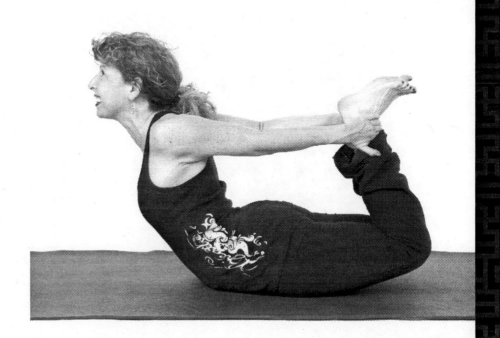

CHRISTIAN YOGA ✣ Postures

Camel - COOL DOWN

STEP BY STEP

1. Kneel on the floor with knees hips with apart and thighs perpendicular to the floor. Shins press firmly into the mat toes tucked or feet flat with toes active and pinky toes pressed into the mat.

2. Inner spiral thighs, firm buttocks but don't harden.

3. Hands rest on the back of the pelvis. Base of the palms on the tops of the buttocks, fingers pointing down. Use hands to lengthen down through the tail bone. Then lightly from the tailbone towards the pubis. Heart lifts and opens.

4. One arm at a time, extend up through the body and then draw hand to the heel.

5. Heart lifts and head drops back. Maintain a relatively neutral position, neither flexed nor extended or allow the head to drop back. One should be able to swallow comfortably.

Benefits

- Stretches the entire front of the body, the deep hip flexor, ankles, thighs, groin, abdomen, chest and throat.

- Strengthens the back muscles and legs.

- Improves posture.

- Stimulates the organs of the abdomen, digestion and circulation.

- Increases spine flexibility.

Contraindications

- High or low blood pressure.

- Migraine.

- Insomnia.

- Serious low back or neck injury.

Common Misalignments

- Feet sickled or asleep.

- Doing outer spiral before inner spiral.

- Lack of shoulder loop.

- Neck is hyper extended.

- Lack of tailbone scooping.

Child - COOL DOWN

STEP BY STEP

1. Kneel on floor.

2. Touch big toes together, sit on heels and separate knees about as wide as hips.

3. Exhale and lay torso down between thighs.

4. Arms extend over the head or alongside of torso.

5. Breathe into the back of the body.

Benefits

- Gently stretches the hips, thighs, low back and ankles.

- Opens upper back.

- Calms the brain and helps relieve stress and fatigue.

- Relieves back and neck pain when done with head and torso supported.

Contraindications

- Diarrhea.
- Pregnancy; keep knees apart.
- Ankle, hip or knee injury: Avoid unless you have the supervision of an experienced teacher.

Common Misalignments

- Feet sickled.
- Shoulders rounded forward.

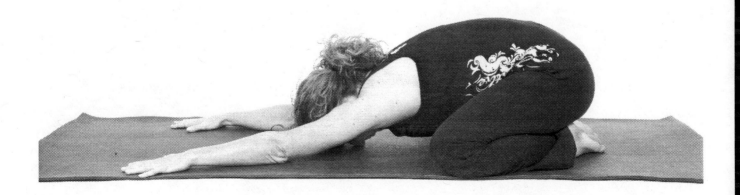

Head Stand - COOL DOWN

STEP BY STEP

1. Start out kneeling on the floor.

2. Place hands on the mat shoulders width apart and then take the crown of the head down 12 inches in front of the hands creating a triangle with the hands and head.

3. Make sure to keep a long gentle curve in the neck when placing head down.

4. Shoulder loop pulling shoulders onto the back and actively extend into the floor with the head.

5. Draw knees up and into body. Knees can rest on the back of the forearms with feet active for Tripod Pose or extend through the heels towards the ceiling coming into the full pose.

6. Body is active and in proper alignment, feet are flexed and toes are active.

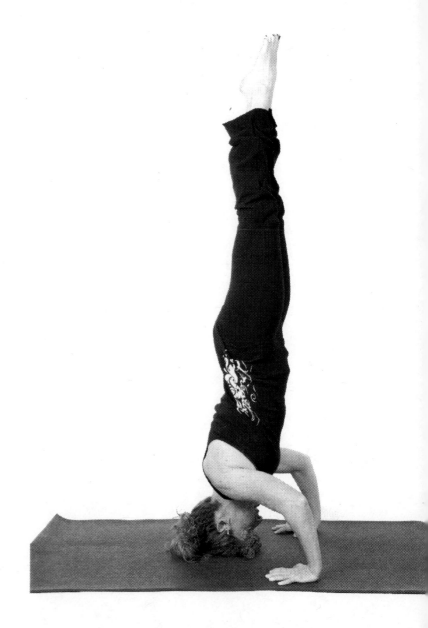

Benefits

- Calms the brain and helps relieve stress and mild depression.
- Stimulates the prostate, pituitary and pineal glands.
- Strengthens the arms, legs, spine and lungs.
- Tones the abdominal organs.
- Improves digestion and circulation.
- Reduces varicose veins.
- Helps relieve the symptoms of menopause.
- Therapeutic for asthma, infertility, insomnia and sinusitis

Contraindications

- Back and neck injuries.
- Headache.
- Heart conditions.
- High blood pressure.
- Menstruation.
- Low blood pressure.
- Pregnancy.

Common Misalignments

- Chin tucked and flattening neck.
- Lack of shoulder loop.
- Legs and/or feet inactive.
- Legs outer spiraled.
- Elbows and/or hands out to the side instead of a stable base.

Incline Plane - COOL DOWN

STEP BY STEP

1. From Staff Pose or Seated Forward Bend pull hands behind hips. Fingers are faced forward and clawing at the mat.

2. Begin to point your toes away from the body.

3. Slowly raise pelvis off the earth and roll your shoulders back till your body is flat and all inline.

4. Feel your gaze go up toward the ceiling and drop your head back. Not too far, make sure you can swallow.

5. Really lift from your heart.

6. On the exhale release back onto your seat.

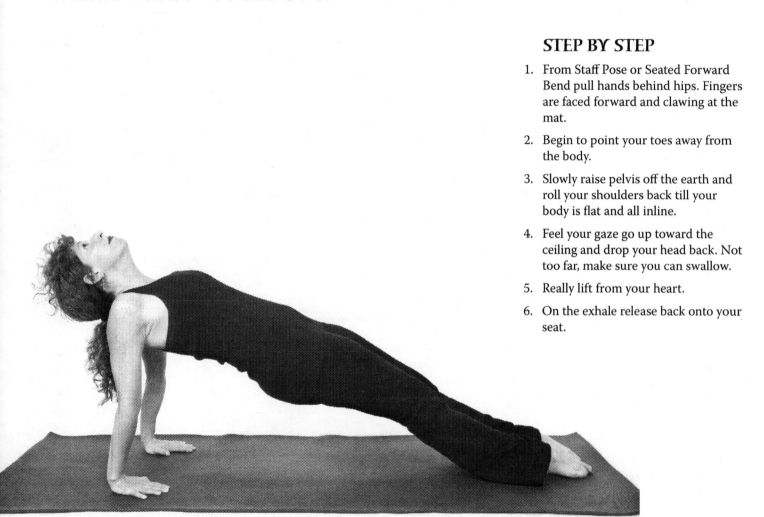

Benefits

- Strengthens and improves endurance of back, leg and arm muscles.
- Opens chest, hips.
- Tones abdominal muscles.
- Increases circulation.

Contraindications

- Shoulder issues
- Wrist issues

Common Misalignments

- Shoulders forward.
- Leg muscles relaxed.
- Legs overly outer rotated.

Locust - COOL DOWN

STEP BY STEP

1. Lie on belly with arms along the sides of torso, palms up, forehead resting on the floor. Big toes towards each other and muscles wrap around the bones and firm the buttocks.

2. Inhale and lift head, shoulders and legs up and away from the floor. Shoulders wrap around the spine.

3. Arms raise parallel to the floor and stretch actively through the fingertips.

4. Gaze forward or slightly upward being careful not to crunch the back of the neck. Keep base of the skull lifted and the back of the neck long.

Benefits

• Strengthens the muscles of the spine, buttocks and backs of arms and legs.

• Stretches the shoulders, chest, belly and thighs.

• Improves posture and lengthens spine.

• Stimulates abdominal organs and circulation.

• Helps relieve stress.

Contraindications

• Headache.

• High blood pressure.

• Serious back injury.

• Students with neck injuries should keep their head in a neutral position by looking down at the floor; they might also support the forehead on a thickly folded blanket. Lift one arm at a time.

Common Misalignments

- Tail lifted.
- Shoulders rounded.
- Head forward.
- Knees bent.
- Toes and/or fingers asleep.

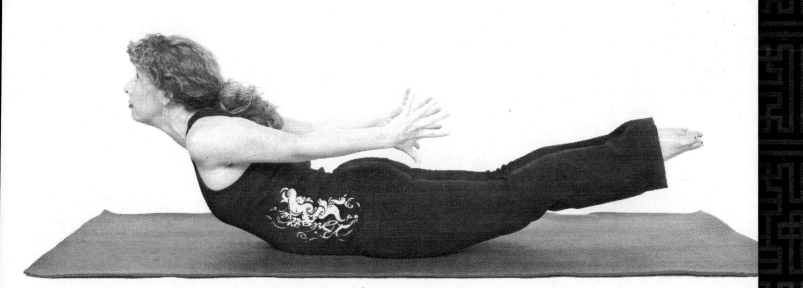

Pigeon - COOL DOWN

STEP BY STEP

1. From Lunge Pose or Downward-Facing Dog draw foot up to corresponding hand setting it down on the mat inside of hand.

2. Walk foot towards the opposite hand and open up letting the knee rest on the mat.

3. Back leg extends from the hip, releases to the mat and remains active. Toes are active as tops of the feet press into the mat.

4. Widen thigh bones and scoop tailbone. Hug legs in (so much so that arms aren't needed for support).

5. Body lengthens through the crown of the head, heart lifts and arms extend over the head. Fingers are active.

Benefits

- Stretches the thighs, groins, abdomen, chest, shoulders and neck.
- Stimulates the abdominal organs.
- Opens the shoulders and chest.

Contraindications

- Stretches the thighs, groins, abdomen, chest, shoulders and neck.
- Stimulates the abdominal organs.
- Opens the shoulders and chest

Common Misalignments

- Back foot sickled.
- Front knees at midline.
- Hips askew, lack of legs hugging.
- Lack of tailbone down.
- Lack of shoulder loop.

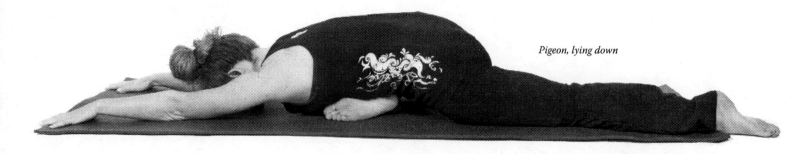

Pigeon, lying down

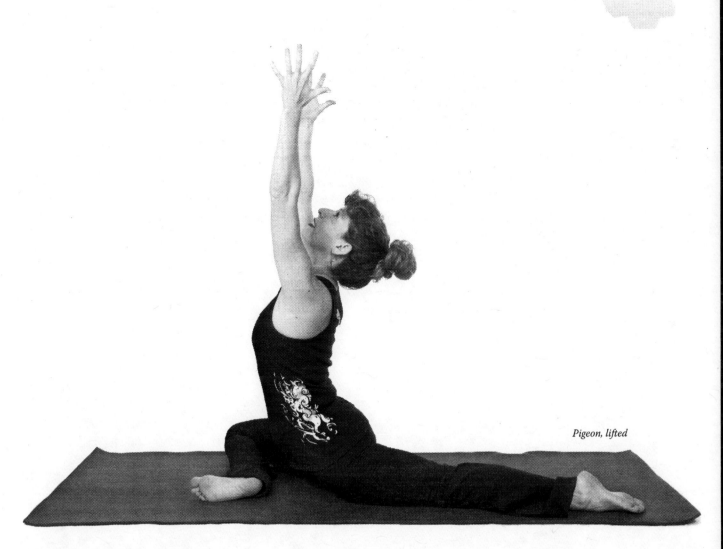

Pigeon, lifted

CHRISTIAN YOGA ✣ Postures

Plow - COOL DOWN

STEP BY STEP

1. From Shoulder Stand bend at the hips and slowly lower toes to the mat, above or beyond the head.

2. Torso is perpendicular to the ground and legs are fully extended.

3. Throat is softened as the chin draws away from the chest. Shoulders and back of the head presses into the mat.

4. Super important to keep chin lifted.

Benefits

• Calms the brain.

• Stimulates the abdominal organs and the thyroid gland.

• Stretches the shoulders and spine.

• Strengthens upper back muscles.

• Helps relieve the symptoms of menopause.

• Reduces stress and fatigue.

• Therapeutic for backache, headache, infertility, insomnia and sinusitis.

Contraindications

- Diarrhea.
- Menstruation.
- Neck injuries.
- Asthma and high blood pressure.
- Pregnancy.

Common Misalignments

- Chin tucked.
- Lack of shoulder loop.
- Elbows out to the side.
- Lack of muscular energy in legs.

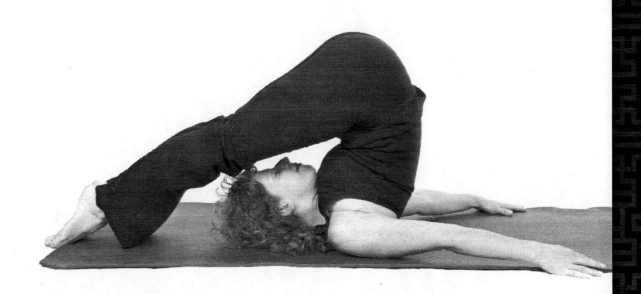

Resting - COOL DOWN

STEP BY STEP

1. Lay down on the back.

2. Feet splay open a little bit wider than hips width apart.

3. Palms are up and resting up by the side.

4. Shoulders draw down away from the ears and relax.

5. Chin rises gently and face softens. Eyes close.

6. Body releases all tension and melts into the mat.

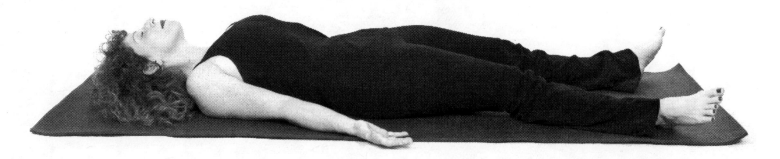

Benefits

- Calms the brain and helps relieve stress and mild depression.
- Relaxes the body.
- Reduces headache, fatigue and insomnia.
- Helps to lower blood pressure.

Contraindications

- Back injury or discomfort; use props like blankets or bolsters.
- Pregnancy; raise head and chest on bolster.

Common Misalignments

- Body is not relaxed.

Seated Wide Leg Straddle - COOL DOWN

STEP BY STEP

1. Start in Staff Pose and then spread the legs a comfortable distance apart.

2. Strengthen thigh muscles while inner spiraling thighs to get the lower back tied in. Shins in and thighs out and work tailbone down.

3. Bend at the hips and lead down with the heart keeping head inline with the spine.

Benefits

- Stretches the insides and backs of the legs.
- Stimulates the abdominal organs.
- Strengthens the spine.
- Calms the brain and nervous system.
- Relieves stress, anxiety, and mild depression.
- Reduces fatigue and insomnia.

Contraindications

- Lower back injuries.
- Asthma.
- Pregnancy.

Common Misalignments

- Lack of muscular energy.
- Legs too outer spiraled.
- Lack of shoulder loop.
- Leading with the head instead of the heart.
- Feet asleep.

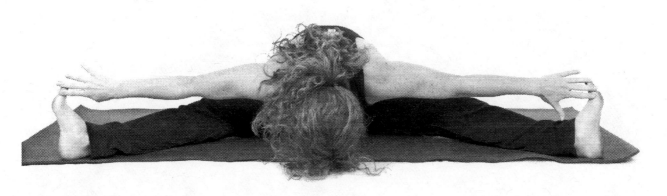

Standing Wide Leg Straddle - COOL DOWN

STEP BY STEP

1. Stand with legs wide apart and feet parallel.

2. Tighten legs by drawing the knee caps up, shins in thighs out.

3. Hands to the hips and hinge at the waist, heart leads down.

4. Fingertips or palms to the mat under the shoulders.

5. Gaze forward and back concaved.

6. You may also grab your big toes.

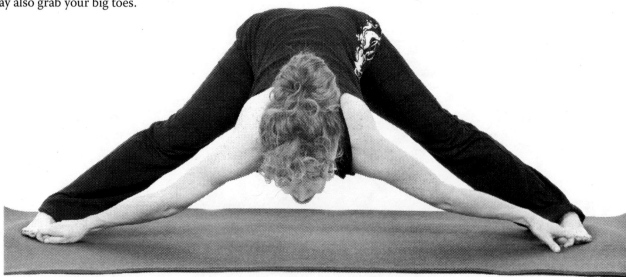

Benefits

- Stretches the insides and backs of Strengthens and stretches legs, feet, ankles, low back and spine.
- Tones abdominal organs.
- Calms the brain.
- Relieves mild backache, headache and sinusitis.
- Improves digestion and circulation.

Contraindications

- Lower back problems; avoid the full forward bend, use props.
- High blood pressure.

Common Misalignments

- Toes turned out.
- Hands dangle with legs straight (use blocks if needed).
- Hyper extended knees.
- Hips behind heels.
- Inwardly rotated upper arms.
- Leading with head instead of heart.
- Lack of shins in thighs out.

Tree - COOL DOWN

STEP BY STEP

1. Start in Mountain Pose and set one foot on the mat with intension. Four corners of the foot on mat and release toes one at the time creating a firm foundation.

2. Draw opposite foot up setting on the mat, shin or upper thigh pressing the heel of the foot into thigh with equal amounts of pressure toes pointing down. Tailbone tucks under.

3. Extend arms up.

4. Do NOT place foot on the knee.

Tree posture, extended

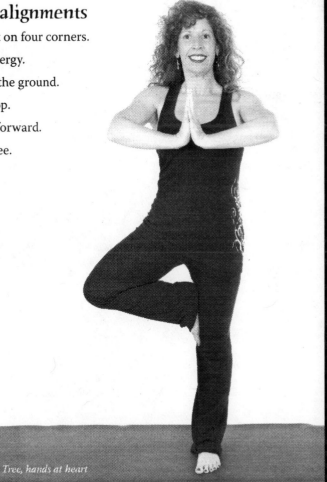

Benefits

- Strengthens thighs, calves, ankles and spine.
- Stretches the groins, inner thighs, chest and shoulders.
- Improves sense of balance.
- Relieves sciatica and reduces flat feet.

Contraindications

- Headaches.
- Insomnia.
- Low blood pressure.
- High blood pressure; don't raise arms over the head.

Common Misalignments

- Foot turned out, not on four corners.
- Lack of muscular energy.
- Hips not parallel to the ground.
- Lack of shoulder loop.
- Standing leg femur forward.
- Foot pressing on knee.

Tree, hands at heart

Wheel - COOL DOWN

STEP BY STEP

1. Come into Bridge Pose, feet actively pushing into the mat, pelvis lifts and buttocks firmed but not hardened. Place hands by the head fingers pointed towards the feet.

2. Firmly press the hands into the mat and shoulder blades against the back and lift up onto the crown of the head. Keep arms parallel and claw at the mat.

3. Press feet and hands into the mat, tailbone and shoulder blades against the back and lift head off of the floor and straighten the arms. Use lots of shoulder loop. Heart leads forward taking pressure off of the legs.

Benefits

- Stretches the chest and lungs.
- Strengthens the arms, wrists, legs, buttocks and abdomen.
- Keeps spine strong and supple.
- Stimulates the thyroid, pituitary, lymph, digestive and reproductive organs.
- Increases energy and counteracts depression.
- Therapeutic for asthma, back pain, infertility and osteoporosis.

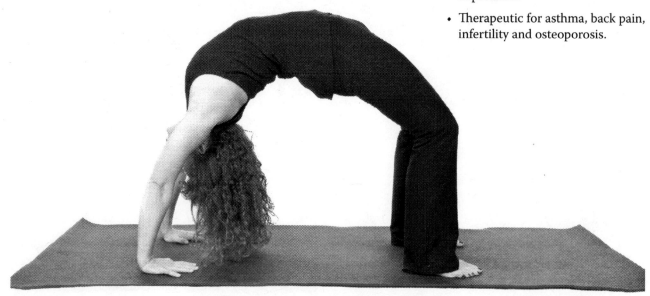

Contraindications

- Back, neck and knee injuries.
- Carpal tunnel syndrome.
- Diarrhea.
- Headache.
- Heart problems.
- High or low blood pressure.

Common Misalignments

- Feet turned.
- Knees out.
- Hands turned in.
- Lack of shoulder loop.

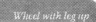

Wheel with leg up

Sun Salutation - PUTTING IT ALL TOGETHER

STEP BY STEP

1. Standing in **Mountain**, raise hands over the head into prayer. Look up.

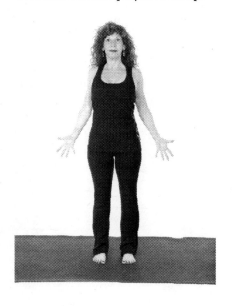

2. Hinge at the waist to the right and take your gaze up to the left. Roll the shoulders back.

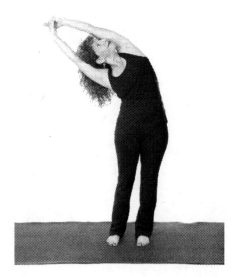

3. Back to center then hinge to the left and gaze to your right. Roll the shoulders back.

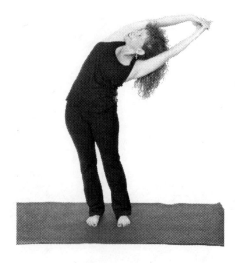

CHRISTIAN YOGA ✢ Postures

6. Bend the knees and jump or walk the feet back to **Plank** pose.

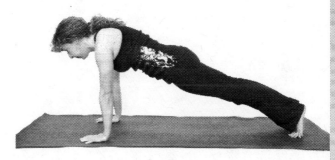

Sun Salutation continues on next 2 pages

4. Back to **Mountain**, then **Open to HIS Grace**.

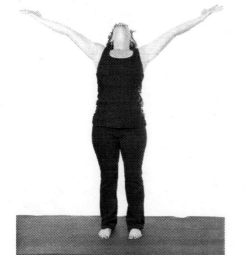

5. Back to **Mountain**, then **Full Forward Bend**.

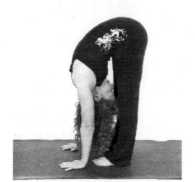

Sun Salutation - PUTTING IT ALL TOGETHER (continued)

8. Inhale **Cobra**.

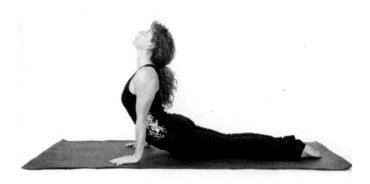

7. Lower down to the **Bottom of a Push Up**.

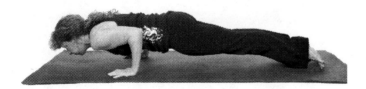

9. Exhale **Downward Facing Dog**.

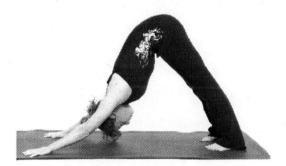

10. **Feet to Hands**.

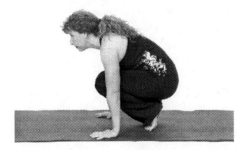

11. **Full Forward Bend**.

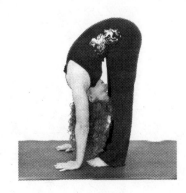

Sun Salutation - PUTTING IT ALL TOGETHER (continued)

12. Back to **Mountain**.

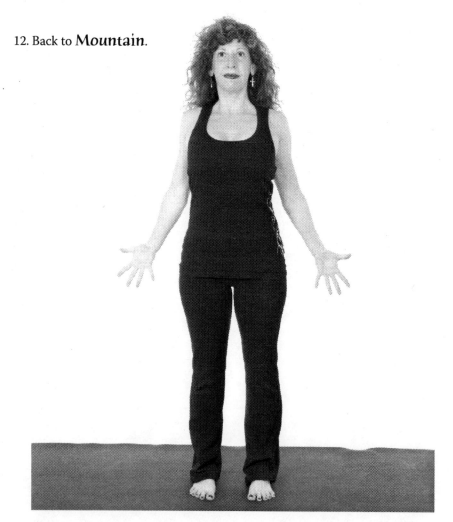

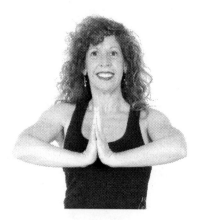

13. Hands rest in prayer at heart's center.

Repeat sequence 5 times.

Benefits

- Builds heat within the body
- Builds strength and flexibility
- Total body workout
- Moves digestive system
- Cardio

Contraindications

- Wrist issues
- Not strong enough yet... come to your knees then lower down to knees belly then chest instead of bottom of a push up.

Common Misalignments

- Leaning forward or back.
- Elbows out as you lower down.
- Shoulders lifted in upward facing dog.

Benediction

A TRAVELER WAS making a trek deep into the jungles of Africa. He hired some local Africans to assist him in his journey. The first day they marched rapidly and made excellent progress. As the second day dawned the tribesmen refused to move and sat resting. The traveler was frustrated with his hired help and found this behavior very strange. When he pressed them to move he was told that they had traveled too fast the previous day and that they were now waiting for their souls to catch up with their bodies.[1]

The LORD bless you and keep you; the LORD make his face shine upon you and be gracious to you; the LORD turn his face toward you and give you peace.
NUMBERS 6:24-26

We trust that you have been encouraged through this book with ways to allow your soul to catch up with your body. We started our journey together with a prayer asking God to bring us to a "spacious place" where we could breathe deeply, move freely and find restoration for our bodies and souls. We will continue to pray for you and your journey in self-care and your Christian yoga practice and that you will find that spacious place where you can meet God and be restored by him.

May you continue to learn the unforced rhythms of grace that Jesus promises to teach us.

May you find life under his yoke to be easy and light.

May your soul be fed with the richest of fare and your body be a temple bringing honor to God.

May you be restored and refreshed daily by God.

May you love God with all your heart, soul, mind and strength and live a life of loving service to those around you.

Finally, dear friends,

Test everything. Hold on to the good. Avoid every kind of evil. May God himself, the God of peace, sanctify you through and through. May your whole spirit, soul and body be kept blameless at the coming of our Lord Jesus Christ. The one who calls you is faithful and he will do it. The grace of our Lord Jesus Christ be with you (1 Thessalonians 5:21-24, 28).

Amen.

---

[1] Story adapted from *Springs in the Valley*, Lettie Cowman, 1946.

Recommended Reading

Celebration of Discipline: The Path to Spiritual Growth
Richard Foster

Soul Feast: An Invitation to the Christian Spiritual Life
Marjorie Thompson

Renovation of the Heart: Putting on the Character of Christ
Dallas Willard

Conformed to His Image: Biblical and Practical Approaches to Spiritual Formation
Kenneth Boa

Satisfy Your Soul
Dr. Bruce Demarest

Thirsty for God: A Brief History of Christian Spirituality
Bradley P. Holt

The Universe Next Door: A Basic Worldview Catalog (4th edition)
James W. Sire

Blah, Blah, Blah: Making Sense of the World's Spiritual Chatter
Bayard Taylor

So What's the Difference?
Fritz Ridenour

Yoga for Christians
Susan Bordenkircher

An Invitation to Christian Yoga
Nancy Roth

Dr. Yoga: A Complete Program for Discovering the Head-to-Toe Health Benefits of Yoga
Nirmala Heriza

About Yahweh Yoga

Yahweh Yoga is an oasis for self-care. Our mission is to serve others by providing outstanding Christian yoga classes, advanced studies, DVDs, books, workshops and encouraging lifestyles that are naturally healthy, fresh and joyful.

Located in Chandler, Arizona, Yahweh Yoga is the first Christian studio in America and is a Christ-centered registered yoga school with the Yoga Alliance®. Come visit our website to order DVDs and find out about our Advanced Studies.

www.yahwehyoga.com